HEART HEALTHY COOKBOOK FOR BEGINNERS:

Discover Delicious Recipes for Lifelong Health - Includes a Low-Fat Guide, Nutritious Snacks, Food Mix Ideas, Expert Tips and a Detailed, Easy-to-Follow Meal Plan

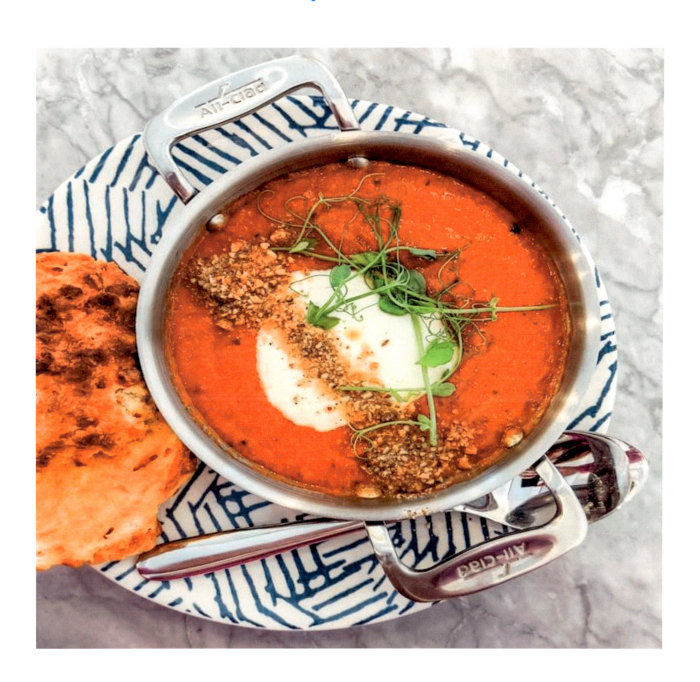

BY JULIETTE GARNISH

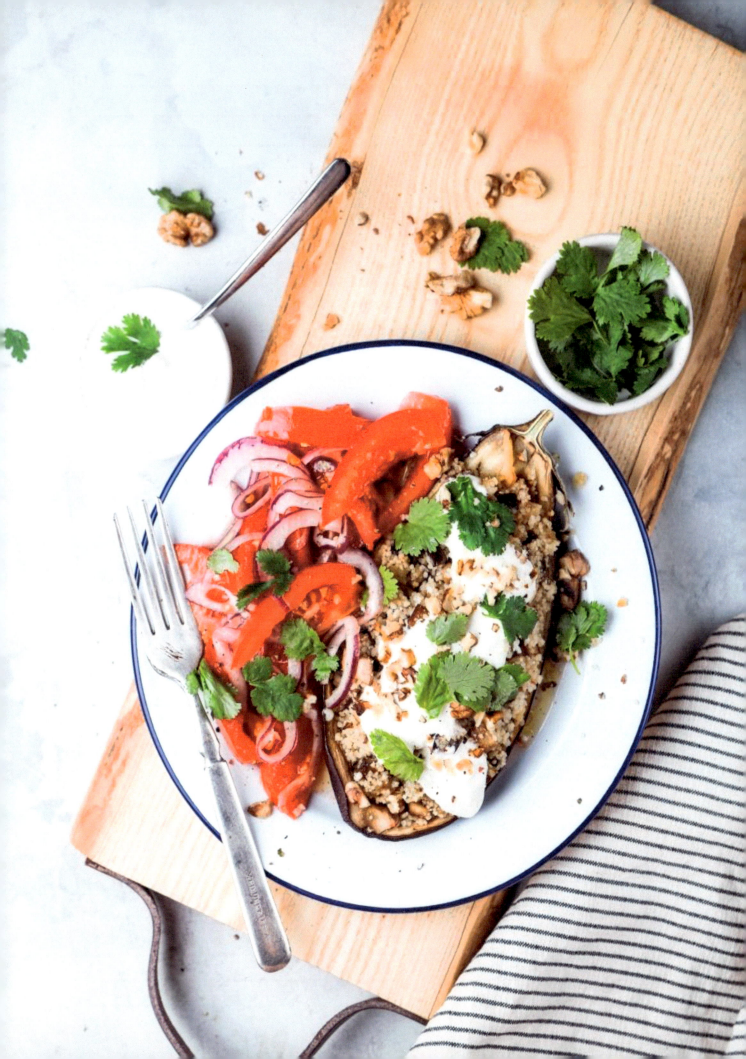

Content

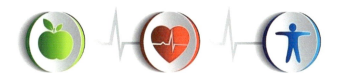

YOUR PATH TO HEART HEALTH FOREWORD

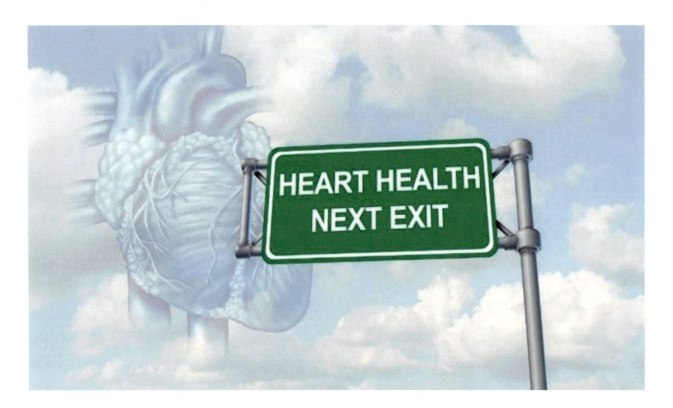

Heart health has become one of the significant public health concerns in the modern world, with millions of people struggling with it daily all around the world. Be it a young professional worrying about having problems when he is your age, a middle-aged adult with the first signs of an unhealthy lifestyle, or a senior who keenly makes efforts to manage irritating conditions, diet has a critical role. This is why I have put together this healthy diet cookbook, accompanied by an extensive collection of delicious recipes designed to promote a healthful lifestyle for the heart. I have created a plethora of dishes that are not just tasty but which meet the unique needs of one or another stratum of the population. There are a large number of busy young professionals who take very little of your time. Middle-aged adults will find nourishing yet light diets rich with cardioprotective nutrients. For our elders, I have designed tasty dishes with attention to balanced nutritional needs and with consideration for possible dietary limitations. But this is much more than just a cookbook. I offer you meal planning, ingredient modifications, and ways to stay motivated while traveling the healthy eating path, whether breaking old habits, dealing with stress, or struggling with a straitened budget. I should be your reliable companion on the journey of changing relationships with food and making the conscious choice of healthy food while experiencing the pleasure of taste. And healthier, happier lives can start with what is on the plate. Join me for better heart health, one delicious bite at a time.

PREFACE

I am thrilled to present the "Heart Healthy Cookbook for Beginners: Discover Delicious Recipes for Lifelong Health." This book is a labor of love, born from a deep personal and professional passion for promoting heart health through delicious and nutritious food. My name is Juliette Garnish, and as a culinary enthusiast, I have always been fascinated by the powerful impact that diet can have on our overall health and well-being.

The inspiration for this cookbook came from my own family's experiences with heart disease. Witnessing loved ones struggle with health issues motivated me to delve deeper into the connection between diet and heart health. I wanted to create a resource that would empower individuals to take control of their health through simple, tasty, and heart-healthy recipes. The journey of researching and writing this book has been both enlightening and challenging. I spent countless hours studying the latest nutritional science, consulting with medical professionals, and experimenting in the kitchen to ensure that each recipe not only supports heart health but also delights the palate.

One of the most rewarding aspects of writing this book was hearing feedback from my relatives and friends — a diverse group of individuals who were eager to improve their heart health. Their positive responses and noticeable health improvements reinforced my belief in the transformative power of a heart-healthy diet. This new edition of the "Heart Healthy Cookbook for Beginners" includes several exciting updates. Based on reader feedback and the latest research, I have added some expert tips, more nutritious snack options, and non-routine food mix ideas to help you navigate your culinary journey. Additionally, I have expanded the meal plan section to provide even more detailed, easy-to-follow plans that cater to a variety of dietary needs and preferences. Writing this book has been an incredible journey filled with learning and personal growth. My hope is that it serves as a valuable tool for anyone looking to improve their heart health and overall well-being. May these recipes inspire you to embrace a heart-healthy lifestyle, one delicious meal at a time.

With heartfelt gratitude,
Juliette Garnish.

INTRODUCTION

You have just come back from your annual visit to your family doctor. The results could be better. Your blood pressure is over the average values, and your cholesterol is beginning to spiral into dangerous territory. This is a wake-up call you cannot afford to ignore. High blood pressure and high cholesterol are considered silent killers. Though they may not seem dangerous at first, they hugely raise the risk of severe cardiovascular events like a heart attack or stroke in case they go unattended. The doctor recommends the worst-case scenario: change your eating habits before this situation goes out of control. But how and where do you begin? Indeed, this heart-healthy Cookbook for Beginners will be your guiding book that will teach you everything you need to know about heart-healthy food and recipes. Should we ban fats altogether? The last time you tried eating fat-free, you were always hungry and annoyed to tears. Are eggs good or bad? You have heard they contain high cholesterol levels but are worth consuming because of the protein they bring. And how can this guilty pleasure of chocolate possibly be? You wish you could keep eating it from time to time. Take a deep breath; this book will be your best buddy. As we wind ourselves through the book's pages, you will discover that eating for your heart does not need to mean depriving yourself and eating tasteless food. Quite the contrary, you will find easy, accessible, and delicious ways to shake up your plate and thus safeguard your precious engine of life. With in-depth, step-by-step recipes, even the most novice cooks will find it easy to start. For all of you who never previously cooked or even think you have no great ideas on the healthy food frontier, such simplicity will kill any doubt about participating in the party. The ready-made weekly meal plan will let you have a well-thought-out menu without the need to wrack your brains hours in advance. But don't you think this book will only give you menus? No, that is not all; here, you will also find tips to help answer all your questions. What food do you need to endow because of its protective effect on the heart?

Which ones, on the other hand, should you cut because of their harmful impacts? No worries, these recommendations will be based on science, not miracle diets or arbitrary no-bans! Can you imagine your blood pressure returning to optimal levels within several weeks, and so do your cholesterol scores? The risk of developing dangerous cardiovascular diseases is drastically reduced. But that is not all! Your everyday energy will also be revitalized. Your body will run like a well-oiled machine by consuming the proper nutrients in adequate quantities. These healthy eating changes to be made for the safekeeping of your heart will not be a chore with a long list of frustrating don'ts. Thanks to this book's delicious recipes and life hacks, this change will happen with all the flavor and conviviality! If once upon a time, having to feed up foods that are too fattening and salty was heartbreaking, now it will be a clear-headed decision for your long-term well-being. The best medicine sources, including the American Heart Association, advise all the suggested hints. For over ten years, I have been helping thousands of patients achieve better cardiovascular health through diet. Well, that means you are in excellent hands here. Ready to put a stop to the risks on your heart health and open a new chapter made up of tasty dishes, practical menus, and newfound energy? Then, let's go on to Chapter 1. Chapter 1 is all about the basics of a heart-friendly diet! Simple steps you need to follow on this path to a healthy lifestyle, one step at a time. The journey starts now.

EMBRACING LIFELONG WELLNESS:
CHAPTER 1: BASICS OF HEART HEALTHY DIET

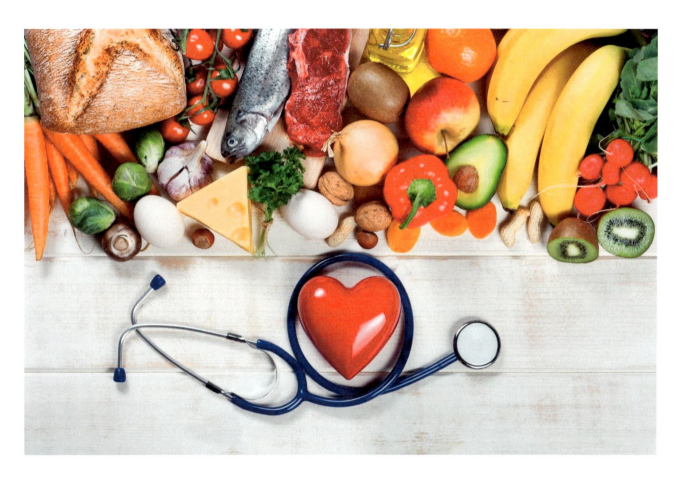

If the heart is happy, then the body will feel healthy. Indeed, the heart is one of the body organs that bring the whole body to life with the help of an individual's circulatory system. A healthy heart beats in a regular rhythm, producing the required strength and distributing the oxygenated blood to all the vital organs and tissues of the body. With the heart acting at this level all the time, the rest of the systems in the human body work perfectly. The muscles are oxygenated, hence nutrients for energy, during movement and involving themselves in physical activities. The brain is well-irrigated and experiences effective concentration, memory, and cognitive abilities. The skin experiences adequate nutritional intake for proper results in being soft, glowing, and healthy. The normal functioning of essential organs like the kidney, liver, and lungs is also supported with blood to carry out the processes of purification and oxygenation. In other cases, atherosclerosis, heart failure, or rhythm disorders weaken the heart, reducing its capacity to pump blood. Such a scenario may give way to poor tissue oxygenation and waste from metabolic processes accumulating in the body, thus resulting in poor functioning of body organs or systems. Contributing poor functioning of the body could result in symptoms like fatigue, shortness of breath, headaches, loss of concentration, or even swelling of the legs. That is why living a life that is friendly to the heart is very important. A healthy diet is a determinant of preserving the vigor and efficiency of this highly appreciated muscle. This energizes the heart, and the whole body functions efficiently, quickly, and in good health. To be more precise, a healthy heart is the key to overall vitality and well-being.

The first fundamental element of a healthy heart diet relies on the type of fat substances in it. It is worth paying attention to good unsaturated fats that tend to have a protective effect, as opposed to harmful saturated and trans fats. Unsaturated fats contain monounsaturated fatty acids (e.g., oleic acid in olive oil) and valuable omega-3 fatty acids.

The latter, mainly in fatty fish such as salmon or mackerel, reduces inflammation and blood clotting. Excellent analysis by the American Heart Association proved that regular fatty fish consumption was related to a 36% decrease in the risk of heart disease. At the same time, however, a high level of research has been taking place over the last four decades that highlighted the harmful effect of saturated and trans fats on "bad cholesterol" or LDL cholesterol levels, which has a central role in coronary heart disease. Analysis of 60 controlled trials, 2549 subjects with average and hypercholesterolemia, mean dose 67 g/d, nut consumption high in unsaturated fats reduced LDL cholesterol 10%. However, the prospective cohort of more than 120,000 women and men estimated that replacing 5% of energy intake from saturated fat with unsaturated fat can decrease the risk of coronary heart disease by 25%. The other nutrient one should be careful about is sodium, essential for heart health. Consumption of vast amounts of salt comes hand in hand with high blood pressure, which weakens the arteries and significantly escalates the risk of cardiovascular events. The World Health Organization postulates that a modest reduction in salt to less than 5g per day would avert 23% of strokes and almost 17% of coronary events worldwide.

The source of proteins is also equally important. Many investigations have confirmed that good sources of proteins, namely legumes, fish, white meats, and low-fat dairy products, are comparably better alternatives when compared with red meat and meat products with a high degree of saturated fat. A large prospective study on more than 80,000 people found that replacing red meat with plant protein sources, such as legumes or nuts, reduced the risk of coronary heart disease by close to 30 percent. Moreover, dietary fiber, especially soluble fiber, prevents the risk of heart disease by its added advantage of enhancing the excretion of LDL cholesterol from the body and controlling blood glucose. A meta-analysis with a comprehensive review that included observational studies and controlled trials showed the risk of heart disease reduced by 9% for every 7g/day increased in the diet of soluble fiber. Foods containing dietary fiber are mainly found in fruits, vegetables, legumes, whole grains, and some seeds. These vital nutritional principles, such as good unsaturated fats, low sodium content, quality lean proteins, and dietary fiber, can be combined into a well-balanced diet to significantly reduce the primary risk for CVD. The heavy support for the most crucial nutritional recommendations regarding long term heart health is witnessed through central, reputable health organizations like the American Heart Association and WHO, as well as many references in scientific papers.

WHAT IS A HEART-HEALTHY DIET?

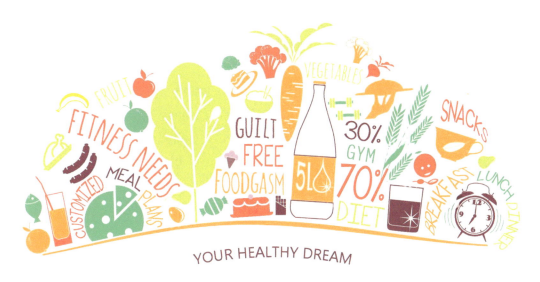

YOUR HEALTHY DREAM

A heart-healthy diet is balanced based on using nutrient-dense foods, restricting unhealthy fats, added sugars, and excessive sodium, and being hydrated to support general cardiovascular health. It is designed to help maintain a healthy weight and decrease the risk of heart disease, stroke, and other cardiovascular conditions while improving overall quality of life. The need for this heart-healthy diet stems from the recent scary statistics. Indeed, globally, over two-thirds of heart disease-related deaths can be attributed to food choices alone. Poor diet and inadequate levels of physical activity are identified as contributory factors to an estimated 6 million deaths annually. According to the American Heart Association, a diet for heart health could cut the chances of deadly heart disease, stroke, and other vascular diseases by up to 30%.

A diet low in fats, high in fruits, vegetables, whole grains, lean proteins, and healthy fats can reduce heart disease by 28%. Fruits and vegetables are the primary sources of vitamins, minerals, antioxidants, and fiber in the diet, which support heart health. A diet consisting of at least five servings of colorful fruits and vegetables can be associated with the reduction of blood pressure, improvement in the blood lipid profile, and heart disease3. For instance, it has been published in the Journal of the American Heart Association that the intake of 1-2 servings of leafy green vegetables a day would reduce the relative risk of contracting heart disease by 11%4. Whole grains contain dietary fiber, vitamins, and minerals that improve blood sugar control and decrease cholesterol. This reduces the risk of heart disease. American Heart Association supports eating at least three daily servings of whole grains to keep the heart healthy. Among great sources of protein that secure your blood vessels and minimize chances for heart disease are poultry, fish, legumes, and low-fat dairy. Among those consuming 1-2 servings of fatty, omega-3-rich fish servings daily, the highest compared to the lowest fish intake quintile, all resulted in evidence for a 15% reduction in developing heart disease, as published in the Journal of the American College of Cardiology.

Healthy fats come from avocados, nuts, seeds, and olive oil. They help maintain an optimum cholesterol level that protects one from heart disease. A study in the New England Journal of Medicine showed through research that people on a heart-healthy diet containing good fats can help decrease their chances of getting heart disease by 30% compared to those on a low-fat diet. Bad fats, added sugars, and added salts must be reduced to minimal consumption if one is striving for a healthy heart. The American Heart Association states that the average amount of dietary sodium consumed daily is less than 2,300 milligrams and no more than 25 grams of added sugars daily.

Besides, an article in the Journal of the American Heart Association stated that lowering daily dietary sodium by 1,200 milligrams could decrease the risks of heart disease by 30%. Hydration is the other aspect of a balanced diet that helps maintain a healthy heart. Dehydration results in reduced blood volumes, an increased rate of the heartbeat, and an increase in blood pressure, all of which finally result in a form of heart disease. The National Academies of Sciences, Engineering, and Medicine advise consuming around 8 to 10 cups of water daily to support overall health.

Therefore, an acceptable diet that has health properties but balances the diet satisfactorily should be considered. This heart-healthy diet is balanced and healthy in a way that supports nutrient density and controls unhealthy fats, added sugars, and excessive sodium intake while keeping a person in a well-hydrated state, promoting overall health. These lifetime recommendations will increasingly reduce one's chances of developing heart disease, stroke, and other cardiovascular diseases.

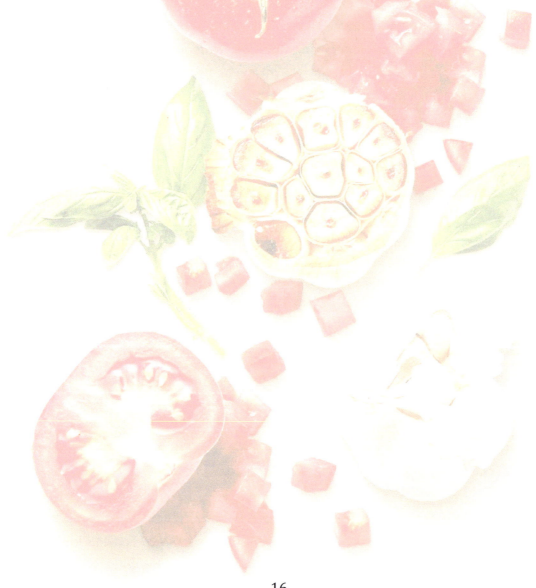

INGREDIENTS TO USE AND INGREDIENTS TO AVOID

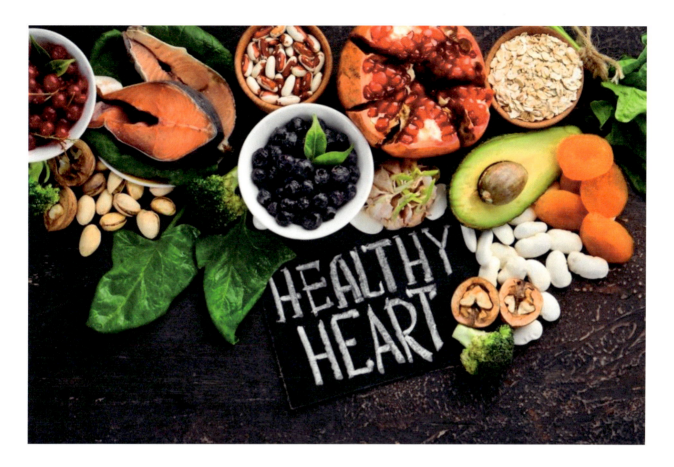

"Everything in food works together to create health or disease. The more we think a single chemical characterizes a whole food, the more we stray into idiocy."

-T. Colin Campbell,

As T. Colin Campbell says in his quotes, focusing on natural and minimally processed foods in one's diet is the key to preserving cardiovascular health. Indeed, a positive approach involves concentrating on what should be cherished in your diet and should be incorporated into it abundantly. Of these precious allies for cardiovascular health are unsaturated fatty acids, which help to control cholesterol levels. On our plate, fiber – those brave warriors against cholesterol. Coming from fruits, vegetables, whole grains, or legumes, they all together make a robust guard for the heart. Here are some of the most essential ingredients that are heart-healthy:

Vegetables and Fruits:

✓ Fresh Vegetables: Tomatoes, cabbage, okra, young soybeans, carrots, Brussels Sprouts, Eggplants, Green beans, brussels sprouts, pumpkins, zucchini, pepper (Green, red, yellow). This variety ensures a diverse and balanced diet, contributing to overall cardiovascular health.

✓ Leafy Greens: Romaine lettuce, spinach, Chinese cabbages, kale, parsley

✓ Fresh Fruits: apples, berries (blueberries, strawberries), oranges, bananas, mango, guava, papaya

✓ Low Sodium Frozen/Canned Vegetables/Fruits

Whole Grain and Whole Grain Products:

Whole Wheat Bread, Bagels, Whole Grain Tortillas
Brown/Wild Rice, Quinoa, Oats
Flakes: oat flakes, barley flakes, kamut flakes
Flours: whole wheat, rye, spelled flour
Crackers: puffed rice crackers, wholemeal rye
Bread: whole wheat bread, whole grain bread
Pasta: whole wheat pasta, legume pasta

Lean Proteins and Alternatives:

Fatty Fish and Seafood: (salmon, mackerel, tuna)
Skinless poultry (chicken, turkey)
Beans, Peas, legumes (beans, lentils), tempeh
Eggs, egg whites, and Tofu
Lean meats: lean beef, veal (Limited quantity)
Limit saturated fat, Sodium, and Sugar

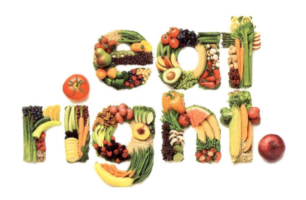

Healthy Fats:

Vegetable oils: olive, canola, rapeseed, flax, walnuts
Oilseeds: almonds, walnuts, hazelnuts, seeds
Nuts and Seeds:
Nut butters: almond, cashew
Nuts (Almonds, Walnuts)
Seeds (Chia Seeds, Flaxseeds, Sunflower Seeds)

Other health foods

Green and black tea (antioxidants)
Spices: turmeric, ginger, cinnamon
Garlic, onion (protective sulfur compounds)
Black cocoa (flavonoids)

Ingredients to Avoid

Knowing what to avoid is crucial in carefully selecting ingredients that will make up a healthy and heart-friendly diet for the long term. As one of the leading global causes of mortality, cardiovascular disease is closely related to everyday diet. Therefore, it is pertinent that we pay attention to the kind of things we eat in our diets every day. We all know that saturated and trans-saturated fat, with excess salt, are enemies of the heart. Overconsumption of these contributes to the elevation of bad LDL cholesterol, blood pressure, and the risk of atherosclerosis—precursors to heart attacks and strokes. Beware of hidden sources of these enemies in informed decision-making. In other words, hyperconsumption of refined sugars and ultra-processed food promotes obesity, type 2 diabetes, and chronic inflammation, which are directly linked with cardiovascular disorders. Knowledge of such ingredients would make avoiding such dangerous dietary pitfalls easier. Here are the essential ingredients that any person wanting to prevent heart issues and maintain a healthy heart should use:

1. Trans fats and saturated fats

Fatty red meats, for instance, lean cuts of beef, lamb, and pig
Processed meats include cold cuts, hot dogs, sausages, and bacon.
Poultry with skin on, for example, chicken or turkey with the skin.
Full-fat cheeses, butter, cream, ice cream—all full-dairy products
Examples are chips, breaded foods, fries, and doughnuts.
Pastries: cream-filled tarts, cookies, and cakes
Nuts, crisps, and nibbles, and snacks

2. Processed Foods and Table Salt

Pretzels, crisps, salted crackers, and aperitif biscuits.
Precooked Foods: Ready Meals and Frozen Dinners
Pickle foods consist of cold meats and smoked or salted seafood and meats.
Salted seasonings: ketchup, mustards, soy sauces, and salty salad dressings
Powdered flavoring for soups and broths

3. High sodium and processed foods

Processed Foods: Packaged snacks (chips, crackers), instant noodles, frozen dinners.
High-Sodium Foods: Canned soups, processed meats (ham, salami), pickles, soy sauce, salted nuts.
Fast Food: Burgers, pizza, fried items from fast-food restaurants.
Bakery Products: Pre-baked bagels, Bread, and Rolls of salted seeds and nuts

4. Sugared Foods and Beverages:

Sweetened beverages include sodas, sweet teas, energy drinks, and fruit punches.
Sweet Treats: Candies, pastries, cookies, cakes.
Containing Sugar: High-Sugar Cereals, Granola Bars.

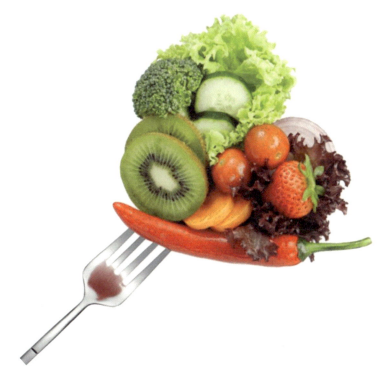

KEY NUTRIENTS FOR HEART HEALTH

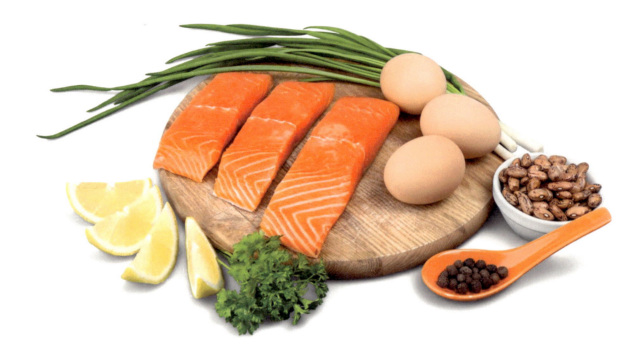

Your health depends on what you eat. Indeed, the connection between diet and heart health couldn't have been better if our hearts had received the needed nutrients. Our heart requires nutrients from our food for energy to keep it beating all day without feeling exhausted since it's a strong muscle that pumps blood throughout our bodies. Besides, these same nutrients play an essential role in helping the formation and functioning of the cells that make up this vital organ; they also control its rate (beating speed) and regulate our levels for either high or low pressures of circulating fluids such as plasma, among others. Moreover, some elements act as antioxidants protecting against free radical damage, which could affect other healthy cells, too, if not neutralized immediately. Any lack of nutrients can lead to malnutrition, which can induce deficiency syndromes (e.g., kwashiorkor and pellagra). Excessive intake of macronutrients can also induce obesity and related diseases. Excessive intake of micronutrients can be toxic. Additionally, the balance of various nutrients, such as the amount of unsaturated versus saturated fat consumed, can influence disease development. The most essential kinds of food elements needed by the heart include but are not limited to:

1. Unsaturated Fats:

Non-fatty fatty acids, also called unsaturated fats, are critical for preserving our heart's health. Unlike saturated fats, they do not increase "Bad" LDL cholesterol levels in the blood. Instead, they can significantly help decrease LDL and growth "correct" HDL cholesterol. W can distinguish between two significant varieties of non-fatty fatty acids:

Monounsaturated fat: These are found in olive oil, canola oil, avocados, and most nuts and seeds. They help lessen inflammation and decrease the risk of blood clots.

Omega-3 polyunsaturated fat: Polyunsaturated fatty acids, particularly omega-3, protect the heart. Those of marine origin have been the most studied. They have anti-inflammatory properties and protect the arteries from atherosclerosis. The recommended omega-3 (AAL) intake is around 1 g per day. Also, the need for omega-3 of marine origin (EPA and ADH) is 500 mg per day. Consuming fatty fish 2 to 3 times per week is recommended to meet these needs.

A. Eating foods wealthy in these non-fatty fatty acids gives our hearts a whole lot of benefits:

They assist in enhancing our "blood lipid level" (a flowery manner of pronouncing fat stability in our blood).

They lessen irritation in our blood vessels.

They help save you "plaque buildup" in your arteries.

They decrease our hazard of having a coronary heart assault or stroke.

In addition, adding a plant source to each can also help meet needs. Good sources of Omega-3 of plant origin are:

Linseed oil and seeds;

Walnut and walnut oil;

Colza oil;

Chia, pumpkin, and hemp seeds.

Oils to use for different types of cooking as part of the cardiovascular disease diet:

Multifunction	Olive oil
Frying	peanut oil
Baking	Rapeseed, sunflower, or olive oil
Flood	Linseed, borage, evening primrose, or hemp oil

2. Fibers:

Fibers found in some plant products like (fruits), (veggies); (cereals) are known carbohydrate molecules that the body cannot break down into simpler compounds. (One) characteristic feature distinguishing them from other types of carbohydrates is that they cannot be digested or absorbed via the bloodstream into the systemic circulation because they lack the necessary enzymes that would have otherwise catalyzed their digestion or hydrolysis processes. Dietary fibers come into two significant classes (either) insoluble (or) water-soluble, i.e., they cannot dissolve in H2O. In contrast, they can dissolve, making something like jelly within human stomachs, hence contributing largely toward lowering lipid profiles through adsorbing what we call (bile salts). This involves restricting bile salts that would have otherwise been re-absorbed in the colon back to their source (the liver) for further processing. This reduces their availability for cholesterol production within the human body, lowering overall blood cholesterol levels. Examples of soluble fibers consist of psyllium, beta-glucan, and pectin. Insoluble fibers, then again, no longer dissolve in water and assist in uploading bulk to stool, promoting everyday bowel actions and stopping constipation. Examples of insoluble fibers consist of cellulose, hemicellulose, and lignin. A weight loss program such as the Heart Healthy diet rich in fiber has numerous benefits for coronary heart fitness. Soluble fibers help decrease LDL (Bad type) cholesterol levels by binding to bile acids and removing them from the body, reducing the amount of cholesterol produced within the liver. An excessive-fiber food plan has also been proven to assist in regulating blood pressure and decrease the hazard of hypertension. Furthermore, fibers have anti-inflammatory properties that can help lessen inflammation in the body, a key threat component for heart disorders. Fibers also function as meals for beneficial intestine organisms, selling a healthy gut microbiome that is important for average fitness, including heart fitness. The American Heart Association recommends that adults consume at least 25-30 grams of fiber daily. Unfortunately, many people fall short of this recommendation, with the average American consuming only around 15 grams of fiber daily. Incorporating more fiber-rich foods into your diet can have a significant impact on heart health, and some high-fiber foods to include in your diet are fruits such as apples, bananas, and berries, vegetables like broccoli, carrots, and Brussels sprouts, whole grains like brown rice, quinoa, and whole wheat bread, and legumes like beans, lentils, and chickpeas.

Here is a table that highlights the most significant sources of soluble fiber:

Food	Portion	Soluble fiber (in g)
Passion fruit	125g	6.5
Black beans	125g	5.4
Beans	125g	5.3
Psyllium	One tablespoon	3.5
Red beans	125g	3
Lawyer	½	2.1
Chickpeas	125g	2.1
Brussels sprouts	80g	2
Coffee	250ml	2
Dried figs	40g	1.9
Flax or chia seeds	20g	1.8
Orange	1	1.8
Yam	100g	1.8
Asparagus	100g	1.7
Turnip	80g	1.7
Broccoli	80g	1.5
Pear	150g	1.2-1.5
Apricots	100g	1.4
Nectarine	1	1.4
Cooked barley	1 cup	0.8
Oat bran	70g	0.4

3. Vitamins and Minerals:

Both minerals and vitamins maintain heart health in complementary yet diversified ways. Foods like bananas, spinach, and sweet potatoes carry a rich amount of potassium, which opposes the effect of sodium on blood pressure. Just like potassium, magnesium found in almonds and flaxseeds plays a vital role in relieving the blood vessels and controlling the heartbeats in the care and protection of the heart. Since vitamins C and E act as anti-oxidants, they are essential in safeguarding the heart's cells from damage. Vitamin B6, B12, and folic acid reduce homocysteine levels in the blood, an amino acid prevalently cited at high levels in those with high risk of heart-related diseases. Food sources of the vitamins comprise citrus fruits, leafy green vegetables, oily fish, nuts, and seeds.

4. Lean Proteins

Lean protein is one major nutrient needed as an amino acid source for repairing and growing body tissues such as heart muscle. It offers all these nutrients, affording high-saturated fat-high protein sources with not all high LDL cholesterol levels. Examples of lean proteins were legumes, such as lentils, chickpeas, and Tofu. Great additions to the diet are lean meats such as skinless poultry and fish, primarily in the form of Salmon and Tuna. Such protein sources are included in daily consumption to achieve sufficient protein content without the related risks of saturated fats. And here is a table that highlights for us the significant sources of healthy proteins for a Heart Healthy diet:

Food	Portion
Chicken breast	100g
Turkey breast	100g
Tofu	100g
Greek yogurt	150g
Cottage cheese	100g
Salmon	100g
Tuna	100g
Eggs	Two large eggs
Quinoa	100g
Lentils	125g
Chickpeas	125g
Almonds	30g
Cottage cheese	100g
Greek yogurt	150g
Tempeh	100g
Edamame	100g
Seitan	100g
Whey protein powder	One scoop

Bison	100g	
Venison	100g	

5. Foods with a low glycemic index

The glycemic index ranks foods according to the increase in blood sugar levels they cause compared to a reference food, glucose. Consuming foods with a low glycemic index can help control blood sugar and cholesterol levels and reduce the risk of heart disease. Here is a table with examples of low—and medium-glycemic index foods. Foods with a low glycemic index and those with a medium glycemic index are preferred.

Categories	Low GI (less than 55) Consume often	Average GI (56 to 69) To be consumed regularly
Bread	Multigrain wholemeal bread	Whole Wheat Rye Pita Bread
Cereals	Oat bran Fiber-enriched cereal	groats
Derivative products	Barley Bulgur Wholemeal pasta al dente Parboiled rice	Basmati rice Brown rice Couscous
Others	Sweet potato Chickpeas Beans Broad beans	Potato Peas

READING FOOD LABELS SMARTLY

When it comes to maintaining a heart-healthy diet, being savvy with food labels is critical. By honing this skill of reading food labels, individuals gain the power to make informed decisions about what goes into their bodies, ultimately shaping their cardiovascular well-being. Understanding the various components of food labels allows for precisely managing vital nutrients that impact heart health, such as fats, sodium, fiber, and sugars. Peering into the world of food labels, the serving size stands out as a crucial focus point. The listed serving size may not align with the typical portion consumed, which can lead to an underestimation of calorie and nutrient intake. For instance, a packet of chips might showcase nutritional data for a serving size of 10 chips, but diving into the whole bag - potentially containing multiple servings - needs a recalibration of the intake of calories, fats, sodium, and other essentials. Minding these serving sizes accurately plays a crucial role in caloric management, given that surplus calories tend to tip the scales towards weight gain, a significant factor in heart disease. Unraveling the interleaved fats on food labels is crucial. These labels typically display total, saturated, and trans fat distinctions. While total fat includes all fat variants in the fare, the tale shifts with saturated fats -commonly found in processed foods and animal products - known to increase LDL cholesterol levels.

Keeping the intake of saturated fats below the American Heart Association's recommended threshold of 7% of total daily calorie consumption is prudent. Steering further away from trans fats is imperative as they have a knack for upping the ante on LDL cholesterol and dialing down HDL cholesterol, paving the road for cardiovascular tribulations. Despite the FDA's crackdown on partially hydrogenated oils, a prime trans fat source, skepticism remains as some processed goodies might still harbor hints of it.

Zeroing in on "0 grams of trans fat" and removing partially hydrogenated oils in the ingredient is essential.

Signaling the importance of sodium content in the heart health arena is also very critical; excess sodium is believed to steer the ship towards hypertension - a prevalent heart disease harbinger. Hence, the recommended cap on daily sodium intake stands at less than 2,300 milligrams, with an ideal ceiling of 1,500 milligrams for most adults, especially those grappling with high blood pressure. High sodium levels are in processed foods, canned soups, frozen treats, and munchies. Poring over labels to manage the sodium content per serving and opting for "low sodium" or "no salt added" picks provides a sturdy grip on sodium consumption. Fiber, especially soluble, is very beneficial for the heart-healthy diet as it helps control LDL cholesterol levels.

High-fiber victuals also help feel full and are pivotal in heart disease prevention. Consuming high-fiber foods like whole grains, culmination, veggies, legumes, nuts, and seeds is crucial for meeting endorsed fiber tiers. Besides, it is vital to monitor sugar consumption to maintain a heart-wholesome weight loss plan, as ingesting too many delivered sugars can bring about better triglyceride tiers and an increased threat of heart ailment. According to the American Heart Association, girls have to restrict their delivered sugar consumption to no more significant than a hundred calories per step per day (about six teaspoons). Men need to aim for no more than 150 calories per day (about nine teaspoons).

Food labels distinguish between general sugars and introduce sugars. People can better control their universal sugar intake by choosing ingredients that might be low in sugars or no longer incorporate sugars. The list of substances offers an in-depth evaluation of the additives of the meal product, arranged via quantity from the highest to the lowest. Identifying hidden assets of bad fats, sugars, and sodium in the components list is essential. Avoiding foods with prolonged lists of surprising ingredients promotes an ample weight loss program in entire, minimally processed foods. Nutrient-dense foods, which give excessive attention to vitamins, which include vitamins, minerals, and different valuable factors compared to their calorie content material, are advocated for maintaining heart health. Foods that might be rich in vitamins A and C, calcium, and iron, however low in calories, fat, and sugars, are taken into consideration to be nutrient-dense. Many studies emphasize the significance of reading meal labels for heart fitness. According to a close study in the American Journal of Preventive Medicine, those who regularly check food labels tend to have a healthier diet and a decreased BMI than those who do not. Another study in the Journal of the Academy of Nutrition and Dietetics found that people who study labels intake less energy, less fats, and more excellent fiber, reducing their danger of heart disease. The Nutrition Facts label, required by the FDA on maximum packaged foods, has been updated to offer more precise information. The revised label, which has become mandatory as of January 2020, features larger fonts for serving sizes and calorie counts and separates brought sugars from total sugars to assist customers in making better picks.

Example:

Let's understand the vital numerical data points and what they mean, using the example of a canned soup to understand nutrition information. The serving size is 1 cup (228g), and that number forms the baseline for all nutrient and calorie information. So, you must adjust your portion size properly.

There are two servings per container, so if you eat the whole can, you consume twice the nutrient and calorie amounts. A serving contains 250 calories, so the entire can be 500 calories—something you need to consider in the context of your daily needs to support weight management and heart health. Total fat is 12g per serving (24g for the whole can); this should focus on minimal saturated and trans fats, but not forget moderate unsaturated fats, which are healthier. Saturated fat is 3g per serving (6g for the whole can); it raises your LDL or bad cholesterol. It should be limited. The trans fats are 0g per serving and should be as low as possible because they are particularly detrimental to heart health. The sodium content is 600mg per serving, and the whole can pack 1,200mg. That's highly associated with high blood pressure, a significant risk factor for heart disease. Opt for lower-sodium options or reduce the portion size. Finally, dietary fiber is 5g per serving so that the whole can have 10g. Dietary fiber contributes to cardiovascular health, so the more of it in your diet, the better it is for a heart-healthy diet.

Numerical Data	Example	Interpretation for Healthy Heart Diet
Serving Size	1 cup (228g)	Establishes the baseline for all nutrient and calorie information. Adjust your portion size accordingly.
Servings per Container	2	It helps calculate the total nutrient and calorie intake if consuming the entire package.
Calories	250 calories per serving	Moderate calorie intake supports weight management and heart health. Consuming the entire can (500 calories) should be considered within your daily caloric needs.
Total Fat	12g per serving	Focus on minimizing saturated and trans fats while ensuring a moderate intake of healthier unsaturated fats. The entire can contain 24g of total fat.
Saturated Fat	3g per serving	Saturated fats can raise LDL (bad) cholesterol. Limit foods with high saturated fat. The entire can contain 6g of saturated fat.
Trans Fat	0g per serving	Trans fats should be avoided entirely as they are harmful to heart health.

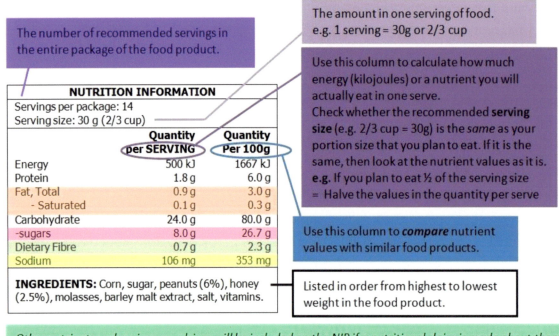

The number of recommended servings in the entire package of the food product.

The amount in one serving of food. e.g. 1 serving = 30g or 2/3 cup

Use this column to calculate how much energy (kilojoules) or a nutrient you will actually eat in one serve.
Check whether the recommended **serving size** (e.g. 2/3 cup = 30g) is the *same* as your portion size that you plan to eat. If it is the same, then look at the nutrient values as it is.
e.g. If you plan to eat ½ of the serving size = Halve the values in the quantity per serve

Use this column to *compare* nutrient values with similar food products.

Listed in order from highest to lowest weight in the food product.

NUTRITION INFORMATION		
Servings per package: 14		
Serving size: 30 g (2/3 cup)		
	Quantity per SERVING	Quantity Per 100g
Energy	500 kJ	1667 kJ
Protein	1.8 g	6.0 g
Fat, Total	0.9 g	3.0 g
- Saturated	0.1 g	0.3 g
Carbohydrate	24.0 g	80.0 g
-sugars	8.0 g	26.7 g
Dietary Fibre	0.7 g	2.3 g
Sodium	106 mg	353 mg

INGREDIENTS: Corn, sugar, peanuts (6%), honey (2.5%), molasses, barley malt extract, salt, vitamins.

Other nutrients such as iron or calcium will be included on the NIP if a nutritional claim is made about them.

To sum up, we can say that the nutritional table helps compare and choose several foods. On the label of prepackaged food, it is mandatory to mention:
Energy value (calories);
The quantity of fats (including the quantity of saturated fatty acids);
The quantity of carbohydrates (including the quantity of sugars);
The amount of protein ;
The amount of salt.

The manufacturer can add:

Monounsaturated fatty acids;
Polyunsaturated fatty acids;
Polyols;
Starch;
Fibers;
Vitamins And Mineral Salts.
Quantities Are Expressed In Grams Per 100 G Or 100 Ml Of Product.

The manufacturer can also express the nutritional values:

As a percentage of intake for a typical adult (reference intakes).
Per serving. However, he chooses the portion size... While some play the game, others use petite portion sizes.

Finally, certain foods do not have to indicate nutritional values   :

Alcohols of more than 1.2%
Unprocessed products that include a single ingredient or category of ingredients,
Water,
Salt and salt substitutes,
Table sweeteners,
Coffee beans or ground,
Infusions (plant or fruit), teas,
Fermentation vinegar,

Chewing gum.

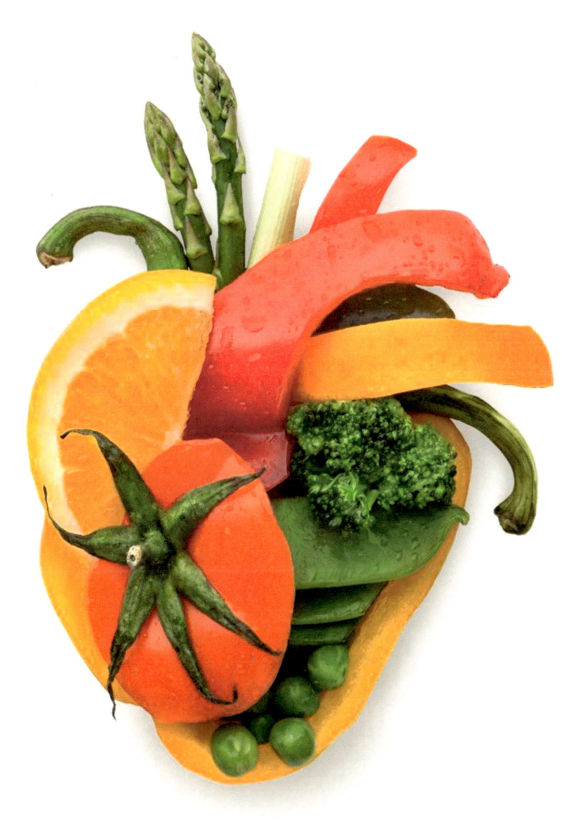

BASIC INGREDIENT SUBSTITUTIONS

Ingredient	Amount	Substitutes
Allspice	1 teaspoon	½ teaspoon cinnamon + ½ teaspoon ground cloves
Baking Powder	1 teaspoon	½ teaspoon baking soda + ½ teaspoon cream of tartar
Baking Soda	1 teaspoon	3 teaspoons baking powder
Barbeque Sauce	1 cup	¾ cup ketchup + 2 tablespoons mustard + 2 tablespoons brown sugar
Butter	1 cup	margarine, vegetable shortening (for baking), oil, coconut oil, nut butter, applesauce, mashed banana, mashed avocado
Buttermilk	1 cup	1 cup milk + 1 tablespoon lemon juice
Chocolate, unsweetened	1 ounce	3 tablespoons cocoa + 1 tablespoon butter or margarine or vegetable oil
Cornstarch (for thickening)	1 tablespoon	2 tablespoons flour or 1 tablespoon instant mashed potatoes
Cream	1 cup	1 cup milk + 1 tablespoon butter
Eggs	1	½ mashed banana or applesauce
Flour, cake	1 cup	1 cup minus 2 tablespoons all-purpose flour
Flour, self-rising	1 cup	1 cup minus 2 teaspoon all-purpose flour + 1½ teaspoon baking powder + ½ teaspoon salt
Herbs, fresh	1 tablespoon, finely cut	1 teaspoon dried leaf herbs, ½ teaspoon ground dried herbs
Ketchup (for cooking)	1 cup	1 cup tomato sauce, ½ cup sugar, and 2 tablespoons vinegar
Lemon Zest (freshly grated)	1 teaspoon	½ teaspoon lemon extract
Milk	1 cup	½ cup evaporated milk
Sour cream	1 cup	1 cup plain yogurt
Soy sauce	1 tablespoon	1 tablespoon tamari
Sugar	1 cup	1 cup coconut sugar
Sugar, brown	1 cup	1 cup sugar + 1 tablespoon molasses
Tomato Juice	1 cup	1 ½ cup tomato sauce + ½ cup water
Wine, red	any amount	same amount of grape juice or cranberry juice
Wine, white	any amount	same amount of apple juice or white grape juice
Yeast, compressed	2/3 oz	1 package (¼ oz) active dry yeast, 2 ¼ teaspoon active dry yeast

CHAPTER 2: BREAKFASTS TO KICKSTART YOUR HEART

2.1.ENERGIZING STARTERS

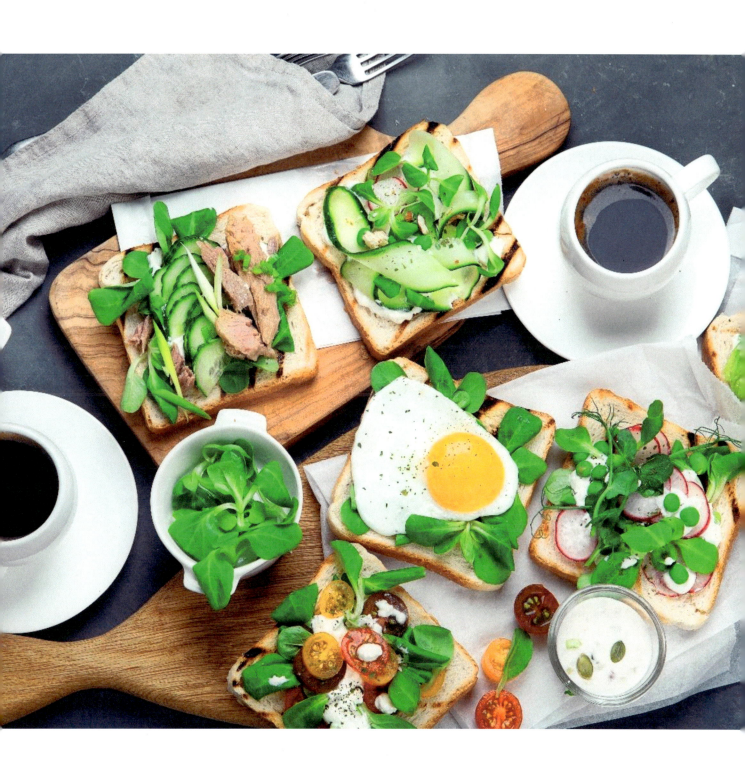

Recipe 1: Cucumber Bites

Prep. time: 10 min | Cook time: 10 min | Serves: 3

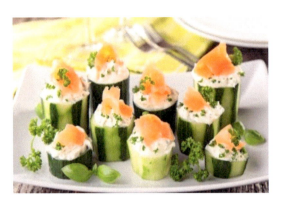

Ingredients:

1 large cucumber, sliced into 1/4-inch rounds
4 ounces cream cheese, softened
2 tablespoons fresh dill, chopped
1 teaspoon lemon zest
Salt and pepper to taste
2 ounces smoked salmon or prosciutto (optional).

Directions:

Mix the softened cream cheese, chopped dill, lemon zest, salt, and pepper until well combined.
Spread a tablespoon of the cream cheese mixture onto each cucumber slice. Top with a piece of smoked salmon or prosciutto (if using). Refrigerate until ready to serve.

Nutrition Information (per serving, without smoked salmon/prosciutto):

Calories: 150, Protein: 4g, Total Carbs: 4g, Fiber: 1g, Fat: 14g, Cholesterol: 30mg, Sodium: 180mg, Potassium: 120mg.

Recipe 2: Deviled Eggs

Prep. time: 10 min | Cook time: 15 min | Serves: 3

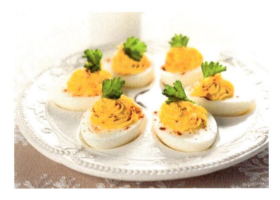

Ingredients:

6 large, hard-boiled eggs
1/4 cup mayonnaise
1 tablespoon Dijon mustard
1 tablespoon fresh lemon juice
1 teaspoon smoked paprika
Salt and pepper to taste
2 tablespoons chopped fresh parsley (for garnish).

Directions:

Peel the hard-boiled eggs and slice them in half lengthwise. Remove the yolks and place them in a bowl. Mash the yolks with a fork, then add mayonnaise, Dijon mustard, lemon juice, smoked paprika, salt, and pepper. Mix well. Spoon or pipe the yolk mixture back into the egg white halves. Garnish with chopped fresh parsley. Refrigerate until ready to serve. Serve and enjoy your starter!

Nutrition Information (per serving):

Calories: 220, Protein: 10g, Total Carbs: 1g, Fiber: 0g, Fat: 20g, Cholesterol: 340mg, Sodium: 220mg, Potassium: 120mg.

Recipe 3: Bacon-Wrapped Avocado Fries

Prep. time: 10 min | Cook time: 1 hour, 20 min | Serves: 3-4

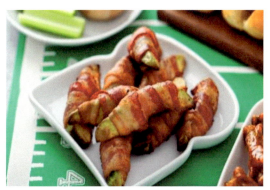

Ingredients:

2 large avocados sliced into wedges
8 slices sugar-free bacon, halved crosswise
1 tablespoon olive oil
Salt and pepper to taste
Ranch dressing or guacamole (for serving, optional).

Directions:

Preheat oven to 400°F (200°C).
Wrap each avocado wedge with a half slice of bacon. Place the bacon-wrapped avocado fries on a baking sheet and brush with olive oil—season with salt and pepper. Bake for 15-20 minutes or until the bacon is crispy. Serve warm with ranch dressing or guacamole for dipping (optional).

Nutrition Information (per serving):

Calories: 320, Protein: 9g, Total Carbs: 10g, Fiber: 7g, Fat: 29g, Cholesterol: 20mg, Sodium: 380mg, Potassium: 480mg.

Recipe 4: Antipasto Skewers

Prep. time: 8 min | Cook time: 10 min | Serves: 3

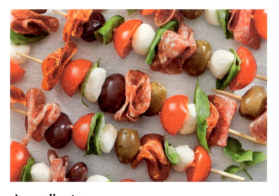

Ingredients:

8 ounces fresh mozzarella cheese, cubed
8 ounces of reduced-sodium salami or prosciutto, rolled or folded
1/2 cup pitted green olives
1/2 cup cherry tomatoes
1/4 cup fresh basil leaves
2 tablespoons olive oil
1 tablespoon balsamic vinegar
Salt and pepper to taste.

Directions:

Grate the mozzarella, salami (or prosciutto), olives, cherry tomatoes, and basil leaves onto skewers.
Drizzle with olive oil and balsamic vinegar.
Season with salt and pepper.
Serve chilled or at room temperature.

Nutrition Information (per serving):

Calories: 380, Protein: 22g, Total Carbs: 6g, Fiber: 1g, Fat: 30g, Cholesterol: 65mg, Sodium: 1180mg, Potassium: 360mg.

Recipe 5: Zucchini Roll-Ups With Goat Cheese

Prep. time: 10 min | Cook time: 10 min | Serves: 3

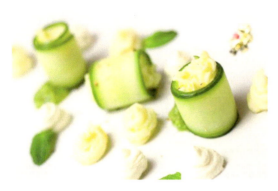

Ingredients:

2 large zucchinis, sliced lengthwise into thin strips
4 ounces soft goat cheese
2 tablespoons fresh basil, chopped
2 tablespoons olive oil
1 tablespoon lemon juice
Salt and pepper to taste.

Directions:

Mix the goat cheese with chopped basil, olive oil, lemon juice, salt, and pepper in a bowl.
Spread a thin layer of the goat cheese mixture onto each zucchini strip.
Roll up the zucchini strips tightly.
Refrigerate the roll-ups until ready to serve.

Nutrition Information (per serving):

Calories: 220, Protein: 9g, Carbs: 5g, Fiber: 1g, Fat: 18g, Cholesterol: 15mg, Sodium: 210mg, Potassium: 290mg.

Recipe 6: Avocado Boats With Tuna Salad

Prep. time: 10 min | Cook time: 20 minutes | Serves: 2

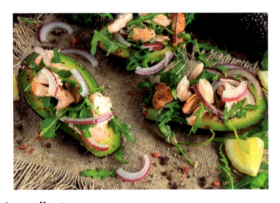

Ingredients:

1 large avocado, halved and pitted
1 (5-ounce) can tuna, drained
2 tablespoons mayonnaise
1 tablespoon diced celery
1 tablespoon diced red onion
1 teaspoon lemon juice
Salt and pepper to taste.

Directions:

Mix the drained tuna with mayonnaise, diced celery, red onion, lemon juice, salt, and pepper in a bowl. Scoop out a little avocado flesh from the center of each avocado half to create a well. Fill the avocado halves with the tuna salad mixture. Serve chilled or at room temperature.
Flavor Variations: Add a kick of heat with a pinch of cayenne pepper, chopped jalapeño, or hot sauce.
Fresh herbs like dill, chives, or parsley can add a wonderful freshness to the tuna salad.

Nutrition Information (per serving):

Calories: 190, Protein: 5g, Carbs: 7g, Fiber: 3g, 4g, Fat: 16g, Cholesterol: 0mg, Sodium: 120mg, Potassium: 290mg.

Recipe 7: Sweet Potato Hash

Prep. time: 10 min | Cook time: 10 min | Serves: 2

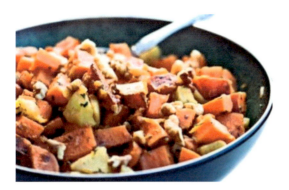

Directions:

In a large skillet, heat the olive oil over medium-high heat. Once the pan starts heating up, add the diced sweet potatoes, the peppers, and the garlic. Once the pan is hot, add the diced sweet potatoes, the peppers, and the garlic, and cook until the sweet potatoes are perfectly tender and browned. While the sweet potatoes are being cooked, heat another skillet with the remaining oil over medium. Once the oil is perfectly heated, add in the onion, salt, and pepper. Cook until the onion becomes soft and transcalent. Combine the ingredients of both the pans and garnish with the green onions. Serve, and enjoy your dish!

Ingredients:

1 Tablespoon of olive oil, divided
1 Medium diced sweet potato
1 Ounce of diced yellow bell pepper
1 ½ Ounce of diced red bell pepper
1 Minced garlic clove
1 Ounce of diced onion
1 Pinch of sea salt
1 Pinch of black pepper, to taste
¼ Large chopped green onion.

Nutrition Information (per serving):

Calories: 101, Protein: 11g, Total Carbs: 10g, Fiber: 7g, Fat: 7g, Cholesterol:130mg, Sodium: 138mg, Potassium: 260mg.

Recipe 8: Spicy Roasted Cauliflower

Prep. time: 10 min | Cook time: 25 minutes | Serves: 3

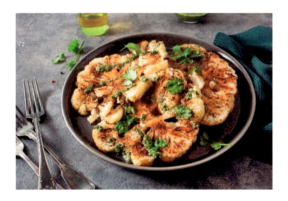

Directions:

Preheat oven to 425°F and line a baking sheet with parchment paper. Cut each broccoli head into halves; then carefully cut each of the halves again. Arrange broccoli on the sheet, season with salt, and drizzle with olive oil. Bake for 20 minutes, then flip and bake for an additional 5 minutes. Meanwhile, heat oil in a frying pan over medium-high heat, add pine nuts, and sauté for 2 minutes, shaking occasionally. Transfer broccoli to a serving platter and sprinkle with pine nuts and chili flakes. Serve and enjoy!

Ingredients:

1 small head of broccoli
1 Tablespoon of olive oil
1 Pinch salt
1 teaspoon vegetable oil, melted
3 TABLESPOON pine nuts
1 Pinch of Chile flakes.

Nutrition Information (per serving):

Calories: 417, 8g protein, 14g total carbohydrate, 6g fiber, 40g fat, 50mg sodium, 630mg potassium.

Recipe 9: Spring Rolls

Prep. time: 10 min | Cook time: 20 min | Serves: 4

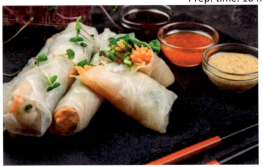

Ingredients:

8 oz shirataki noodles or zucchini noodles
8 oz shredded carrots Shredded 1 cup
Cabbage
1/2 cup red bell pepper, julienned
1/2 cup cucumber, sliced thin
1/4 c fresh mint leaves, chopped
1/4 cup fresh cilantro, chopped
8 oz shelled and deveined shrimp, cooked
8-10 whole-grain wraps, think lettuce,
cabbage,2 tablespoons of rice vinegar 1
tablespoon of low-sodium tamari or coconut
aminos 1 teaspoon of sesame oil 1 garlic
clove, minced Lime wedges for serving.

Directions:

If using shirataki noodles, rinse and drain well. If using zucchini noodles, make them as you like.
In a big bowl, mix the noodles, shredded carrot, cabbage, bell pepper, cucumber, mint, cilantro, and shrimp (if using). Whisk together the rice vinegar, low-sodium tamari (or coconut), sesame oil, and minced garlic in a small bowl. Drizzle the dressing over the noodle mixture and very carefully toss together. Scoop about 1/4 cup of the noodle mixture onto the lower third of a wrap (lettuce, cabbage) Finally, roll the bottom edge over the top of the filling, tuck in the ends, and tightly roll it up into a cylinder. Repeat with the remaining wraps and filling. Serve the spring rolls with lime wedges for squeezing over the top.

Nutrition Information (per serving):

Calories: 120, Protein: 4g, Total Carbs: 12g, Fiber: 4g, Fat: 7g, Cholesterol: 0mg, Sodium: 120mg, Potassium: 400mg

Recipe 10: Stuffed Grape Leaves

Prep. time: 20 min | Cook time: 10 min | Serves: 4

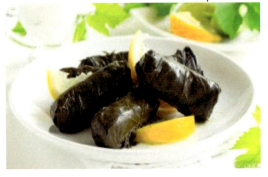

Ingredients:

1 jar grape leaves, rinsed
1 cup brown rice, cooked
1/2 cup of tomatoes, chopped
1/4 cup fresh parsley, chopped
1/4 cup fresh mint, chopped
1 tablespoon olive oil
The juice of 1 lemon
Black pepper to taste.

Directions:

Combine cooked brown rice, chopped herbs, and diced tomatoes in a bowl. Mix well with olive oil, black pepper, and fresh lemon juice. Lay a grape leaf flat, vein side down. Place a spoonful of the rice mixture on the stem end, fold the stem over the filling, fold in the sides, and roll into a cylinder. Repeat with remaining leaves and filling. Arrange stuffed grape leaves on a dish, cover, and refrigerate until serving. Serve chilled, with garnish or extra lemon wedges if desired.

Nutrition Information (per serving, about 3 stuffed grape leaves):

Calories: 150, 3g protein, 28g total carbohydrate, 3g fiber, 4g fat, 20mg sodium, 280mg potassium.

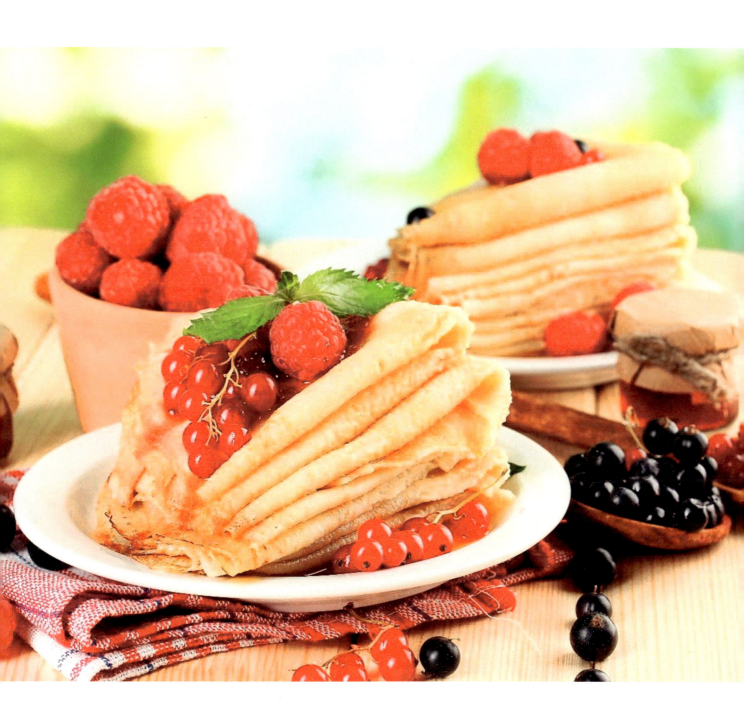

Recipe 11: Cinnamon Pancakes

Prep. time: 10 min | Cook time: 10 min | Serves: 3

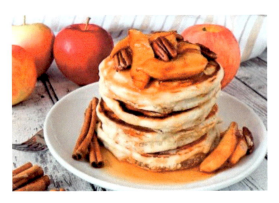

Ingredients:

½ cup of low-carb flour blend (together with almond flour or coconut flour)
½ cup of mascarpone or cream cheese (at room temperature)
3 large eggs, 2 tablespoons of granulated erythritol or monk fruit sweetener
1 teaspoon of baking powder
Toppings of your desire (e.g., berries, sugar-loose syrup, whipped cream, nuts).

Directions:

Whisk together the low-carb flour blend, sweetener, and baking powder in a large bowl. Create a well in the center, crack the eggs, and whisk to incorporate the dry ingredients. Add mascarpone or cream cheese and blend until smooth.

Heat a non-stick skillet over medium heat and lightly grease with butter or oil. Pour 1/4 cup of batter for each pancake, cooking until bubbles form (2-3 minutes). Flip and cook for another 1-2 minutes until golden brown. Repeat with remaining batter, greasing as needed. Serve warm with your favorite toppings.

Nutrition Information:

Calories: 275, 11g protein, 6g carbohydrates, 22g fat, 3g fiber, 0mg cholesterol, 180mg sodium, 209g potassium.

Recipe 12: Breakfast Strata

Prep. time: 15 min | Cook time: 70-80 min | Serves: 4

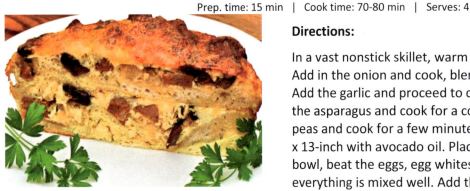

Ingredients:

1 tablespoon of avocado oil, 1 large onion, diced (approximately 2 cups), 2 cloves garlic, minced
1/2 bunch asparagus (around 1/2 pound), trimmed and cut into 1-inch (2.5-cm) pieces
1 ½ cups of green peas
1 whole-wheat baguette, cut into 1-inch pieces, 6 Large eggs, 10 egg whites
2 cups of coconut milk 1 tablespoon of Dijon mustard 1/4 cup of grated Parmesan cheese
2 oz (60 g) part-skim mozzarella cheese
1 Large carrot, 1 cup of sundried chopped tomatoes, 1 tablespoon of dried tarragon
1/2 teaspoon of ground dark pepper.

Directions:

In a vast nonstick skillet, warm the oil over medium-high heat. Add in the onion and cook, blending for around 3 minutes. Add the garlic and proceed to cook for about 1 minute. Add the asparagus and cook for a couple of minutes. Add in the peas and cook for a few minutes. Coat a baking dish of about 9 x 13-inch with avocado oil. Place the chopped bread in a large bowl, beat the eggs, egg whites, drain, and mustard until everything is mixed well. Add the mixture of vegetables, cheeses, carrots, sun-dried tomatoes, tarragon, and pepper, blending well.
Pour the blend over the bread, cover it with plastic wrap, and refrigerate overnight or at least 8 hours. Remove the strata from the fridge and let it sit at room temperature while you preheat the stove to 350 °F (180 °C). Don't keep at room temperature for more than 20 minutes. Bake for about 70 to 80 minutes.

Nutritional Information:

Calories: 240, 19g protein, 23g carbohydrates, 8g fat, 6g fiber, 12mg cholesterol, 280mg sodium, 220g potassium.

Recipe 13: Almond Chia Pudding

Prep. time: 15 min | Cook time: 10 min | Serves: 2-3

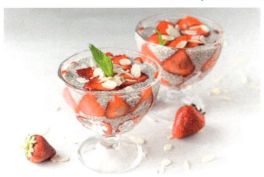

Ingredients:

1/four cup chia seeds
1 cup of unsweetened almond milk
1 teaspoon vanilla extract
1/4 teaspoon of ground cinnamon
¼ cup of berries (blueberries, raspberries, or strawberries)
1 tablespoon of chopped nuts (almonds, pecans, or walnuts) (optional)
1 tablespoon of Stevia or a different sugar alternative to taste

Directions:

Whisk together chia seeds, almond milk, vanilla extract, and cinnamon in a jar or bowl. Let sit down for at least 15 minutes or overnight for a thicker pudding. Top with sparkling berries and nuts (non-obligatory). Sweeten with stevia to taste if desired. Serve and enjoy your breakfast!

Variations:

Use coconut milk or heavy cream for a more decadent pudding. Add a scoop of unsweetened protein powder Substitute berries with chopped fruit like mango or peaches.

Tips:

Soaking the chia seeds daily creates a thicker, creamier pudding.

Nutrition Information:

Calories: 280, 6g protein, 7g carbohydrates, 18g fat, 11g fiber, 7mg cholesterol, 30mg sodium, 180g potassium.

Recipe 14: Coconut Flour Waffles

Prep. time: 10min | Cook time: 15 min | Serves: 2-3

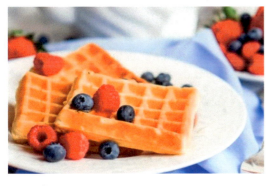

Ingredients:

1/2 cup coconut flour
1/4 cup melted almond butter or avocado oil
4 large eggs
1/4 cup unsweetened almond milk
2 tablespoons erythritol or monk fruit sweetener
1 teaspoon baking powder
1/2 teaspoon vanilla extract
Pinch of salt.

Directions:

Whisk together the coconut flour, baking powder, erythritol, and salt in a bowl.
Beat the eggs in a separate bowl, then add the melted butter, almond milk, and vanilla extract.
Slowly add the dry ingredients to the wet ingredients and mix until well combined.
Preheat a waffle iron and lightly grease with butter or cooking spray. Pour the batter onto the hot waffle iron and cook until golden brown, about 5-7 minutes.
Serve hot with your favorite toppings, such as sugar-free syrup, berries, or whipped cream.

Nutrition Information:

Calories: 290, 7g protein, 7g carbohydrates, 15g fat, 10g fiber, 6mg cholesterol, 45mg sodium, 190g potassium.

Recipe 15: Salmon Scramble

Prep. time: 10 min | Cook time: 10 min | Serves: 2

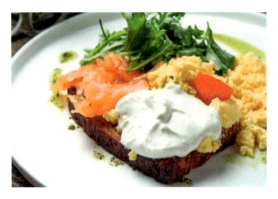

Ingredients:

4 large eggs
1 tablespoon olive oil or avocado oil (instead of butter to reduce saturated fat)
4 oz smoked salmon or cooked salmon, flaked
2 oz low-fat cream cheese
1 tablespoon fresh dill, chopped.

Directions:

Crack the eggs right into a bowl and whisk till blended.
Melt the butter in a skillet over medium heat.
Pour inside the eggs and gently push/pull with a spatula to scramble.
When eggs are still moist, stir in the salmon, cream cheese, and dill.
Remove from heat when the cream cheese is melted and the eggs are set, but they will remain wet.
Season with salt and pepper.

Nutrition Information:

Calories 345, Protein 22g, Total Carbs 13g, Fiber 5g, Fat 24g, Cholesterol 240mg, Sodium 430mg, Potassium 230mg.

Recipe 16: Cauliflower Hash Browns

Prep. time: 10 min | Cook time: 12min | Serves: 4

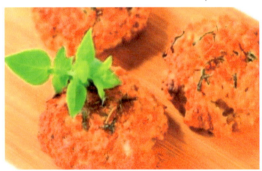

Ingredients:

1 medium head of cauliflower, grated or finely chopped
2 large eggs, beaten
1/4 cup grated Parmesan cheese
2 tablespoons almond flour
1 teaspoon garlic powder
Salt and pepper to taste
2 tablespoons butter or olive oil

Directions:

Grate or finely chop the cauliflower to resemble rice.
Mix the cauliflower rice with beaten eggs, Parmesan cheese, almond flour, garlic powder, salt, and pepper in a bowl. Heat butter or olive oil in a large skillet over medium heat. Scoop the cauliflower mixture into the skillet and flatten into rounds or patties.
Cook for 4-5 minutes per side or until golden brown and crispy. Serve hot and enjoy!

Nutrition Information (per serving):

Calories: 200, Protein: 9g, Total Carbs: 7g, Fiber: 3g, Fat: 16g, Cholesterol: 125mg, Sodium: 350mg, Potassium: 360mg.

Recipe 17: Coconut Yogurt Parfait

Prep. time: 10 min | Cook time: 5 min | Serves: 2

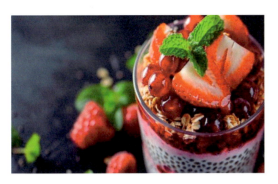

Ingredients:

1 cup unsweetened coconut yogurt
1/4 cup fresh raspberries
1/4 cup fresh blueberries
2 tablespoons chia seeds
2 tablespoons sliced almonds
1 tablespoon unsweetened shredded coconut
1 tablespoon erythritol or monk fruit
sweetener (optional).

Directions:

Layer the coconut yogurt, berries, chia seeds, almonds, and coconut in glasses.
Sweeten with erythritol if desired.
Refrigerate until ready to serve or enjoy immediately.

Variations:

Use different berries or chopped nuts.
Substitute Greek yogurt for coconut yogurt.
Add a dollop of nut butter or sugar-free jam.

Tips:

Make parfaits ahead for a grab-and-go breakfast.
Use mason jars or to-go cups for easy transport.

Nutrition Information (per muffin):

Calories 280, Protein 6g, Total Carbs 12g, Fiber 8g, 4g, Fat 23g, Cholesterol 0mg, Sodium 35mg, Potassium 280mg.

Recipe 18: Smoked Salmon Frittata

Prep time: 10 min | Cook time: 30 min | Serves: 4

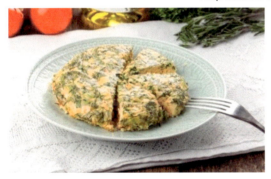

Ingredients:

6 large eggs
1/2 cup heavy cream
1/2 cup crumbled feta cheese
2 tablespoons fresh dill, chopped
1/2 teaspoon salt
1/4 teaspoon black pepper
4 ounces smoked salmon, chopped
Butter or cooking spray (to grease the baking dish).

Directions:

Preheat oven to 350°F.
Whisk eggs, cream, feta, dill, salt and pepper.
Stir in salmon. Grease a baking dish and pour in the egg mixture. Bake 20-25 mins until center is set.
Let cool slightly before slicing.

Variations:

Add sautéed spinach or mushrooms.
Substitute goat cheese for feta.
Use cooked bacon instead of smoked salmon.

Tips:

It can be made ahead and reheated.
Great for meal prep - refrigerate well.

Nutrition Information (per serving):

Calories 290, Protein 21g, Total Carbs 2g, Fiber 0g, s 2g, Fat 22g, Cholesterol 435mg, Sodium 186mg, Potassium 260mg.

Recipe 19: Shakshuka

Prep time: 9 min | Cook time: 10min | Serves: 3-4

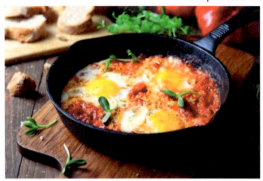

Ingredients:

1 tablespoon of olive oil
1 onion chopped
3 garlic, minced
1 red bell pepper, diced
1 teaspoon smoked paprika
1 teaspoon cumin
1/4 teaspoon cayenne pepper (optional for heat)
1 (28 oz) can crushed tomatoes, low sodium
6 large eggs
1/4 cup chopped fresh parsley
Salt and black pepper to taste.

Directions:

Heat the olive oil in a large ovenproof skillet over medium heat. Add chopped onions and sauté until transparent for 2-3 minutes. Add the minced garlic and diced bell pepper; cook another 2 minutes.

Add the smoked paprika, cumin, and the cayenne pepper if using. Sauté for 1 minute until fragrant.

Add the low-sodium crushed tomatoes, allowing the mixture to simmer. Make a well into the tomato mixture and crack the eggs directly into each of the wells. Cover the skillet and let the eggs cook for 5-7 minutes, or until the whites are set and the yolks are cooked to your desired doneness.

Take off the heat and garnish with chopped fresh parsley. Taste and season with salt and black pepper.

Nutrition Information (per serving, about 1/4 of the recipe):

Calories: 220, Protein: 12g, Total Carbs: 18g, Fiber: 4g, Fat: 11g, Cholesterol: 185mg, Sodium: 200mg, Potassium: 650mg.

Recipe 20: Mascarpone & Berries Toast

Prep. time: 10 min | Cook time: 5 min | Serves: 2-3

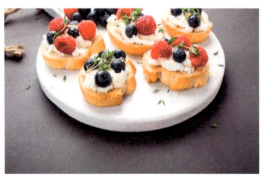

Ingredients:

4 slices keto-friendly bread (like almond flour or coconut flour bread)
1/2 cup mascarpone cheese
1/2 cup fresh mixed berries (like strawberries, blueberries, raspberries)
1 tablespoon erythritol or monk fruit sweetener (optional)
1 teaspoon vanilla extract
1 tablespoon chopped nuts (like almonds or pecans) (optional).

Directions:

Toast the keto bread slices until golden brown.

In a small bowl, mix the mascarpone cheese, vanilla extract, and sweetener (if using). Spread the mascarpone mixture evenly over the toasted bread slices. Top with fresh berries and chopped nuts (if using).

Variations:

Use ricotta or cream cheese instead of mascarpone. Drizzle with sugar-free syrup or sprinkle with cinnamon. Top with a dollop of unsweetened whipped cream.

Tips:

Let the mascarpone cheese come to room temperature for easier spreading.

Use frozen berries if fresh ones are not in season.

Nutrition (per serving):

Calories 320, Protein 12g, Total Carbs 12g, Fiber 5g, Fat 25g, Cholesterol 60mg, Sodium 220mg, Potassium 180mg.

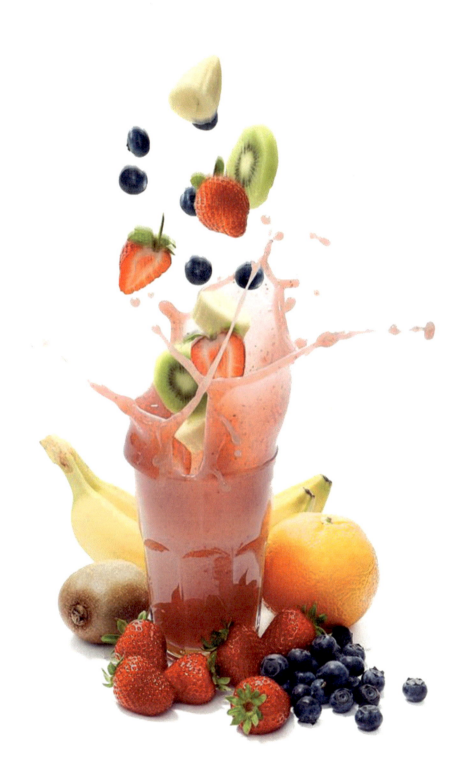

Recipe 21: Spinach And Chia Smoothie

Prep. time: 5 min | Cook time: 5 min | Serves: 2

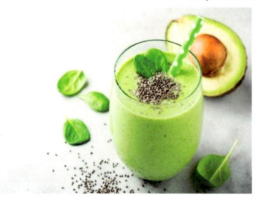

Ingredients:

1 cup unsweetened almond milk
1 cup fresh spinach
1/2 avocado
1/4 cup full-fat coconut milk
1 tablespoon almond butter
1 tablespoon chia seeds
1 tablespoon erythritol (optional)
1/2 teaspoon vanilla extract.

Directions:

Add all ingredients to a blender and blend until smooth.
Adjust sweetness with erythritol if desired.
Pour into a glass.
Serve and enjoy your smoothie!

Variations:

Use coconut milk instead of almond milk.
Add a scoop of vanilla or chocolate keto protein powder.
Substitute kale or romaine lettuce for spinach.

Tips:

Add a handful of ice cubes for a thicker, frosty texture.
Use frozen spinach or avocado for an extra creamy smoothie.

Nutrition Information (per serving):

Calories 420, Protein 9g, Total Carbs 12g, Fiber 9g, 3g, Fat 38g, Cholesterol 0mg, Sodium 160mg, Potassium 380mg.

Recipe 22: Peanut Butter Smoothie

Prep. time: 5 min | Cook time: 5 min | Serves: 2

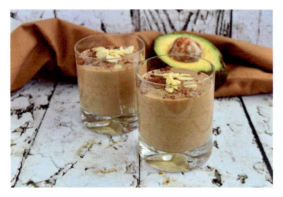

Ingredients:

1 cup unsweetened almond milk
1/2 cup frozen mixed berries
1/4 cup full-fat Greek yogurt
2 tablespoons almond butter
1 tablespoon chia seeds
1 tablespoon erythritol (optional)
1/2 teaspoon vanilla extract.

Directions:

Add all ingredients to a blender and blend until smooth.
Adjust sweetness with erythritol if desired.
Pour into a glass.
Serve and enjoy your smoothie!

Variations:

Use coconut milk instead of almond milk.
Add a scoop of vanilla or strawberry keto protein powder.
Substitute different berries like raspberries or blackberries.

Nutrition Information (per serving):

Calories 410, Protein 14g, Total Carbs 11g, Fiber 7g, 3.4g, Fat 35g, Cholesterol 0mg, Sodium 240mg, Potassium 400mg.

Recipe 23: Berry Smoothie

Prep. time: 5 min | Cook time: 5 min | Serves: 2

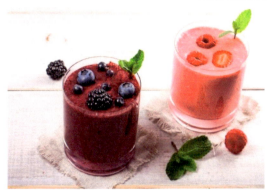

Ingredients:

1 cup unsweetened almond milk
1/2 cup frozen mixed berries
1/4 cup full-fat Greek yogurt
2 tablespoons almond butter
1 tablespoon chia seeds
1 tablespoon erythritol (optional)
1/2 teaspoon vanilla extract.

Directions:

Add all ingredients to a blender and blend until smooth.
Adjust sweetness with erythritol if desired.
Pour into a glass.
Serve and enjoy your smoothie!

Variations:

Use coconut milk instead of almond milk.
Add a scoop of vanilla or strawberry keto protein powder.
Substitute different berries like raspberries or blackberries.

Tips:

Use frozen berries for a thicker, frosty texture.
Add a handful of greens like spinach or kale for extra nutrients.

Nutrition Information (per serving):

Calories 370, Protein 13g, Total Carbs 14g, Fiber 8g, 6g, Fat 38g, Cholesterol 10mg, Sodium 180mg, Potassium 370mg.

Recipe 24: Coconut Smoothie

Prep. time: 5 min | Cook time: 5 min | Serves: 2

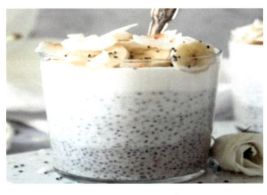

Ingredients:

1 cup unsweetened coconut milk
1/4 cup full-fat Greek yogurt
2 tablespoons unsweetened shredded coconut
1 tablespoon chia seeds
1 tablespoon erythritol (optional)
1/2 teaspoon vanilla extract.

Directions:

Add all ingredients to a blender and blend until smooth.
Adjust sweetness with erythritol if desired.
Pour into a glass.
Serve and enjoy!

Variations:

Use almond milk instead of coconut milk.
Add a scoop of vanilla or coconut keto protein powder.
Mix in a tablespoon of unsweetened cocoa powder.

Tips:

Use coconut cream instead of yogurt for a richer texture.
Toast the shredded coconut for extra flavor.

Nutrition Information (per serving):

Calories 330, Protein 7g, Total Carbs 13g, Fiber 6.4g, 6g, Fat 28g, Cholesterol 10mg, Sodium 100mg, Potassium 320mg.

Recipe 25: Cocoa Avocado Smoothie

Prep. time: 5 min | Cook time: 10 min | Serves: 2

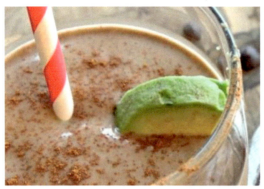

Ingredients:

1 cup unsweetened almond milk
1/2 avocado
2 tablespoons unsweetened cocoa powder
2 tablespoons almond butter
1 tablespoon chia seeds
1 tablespoon erythritol (optional)
1/2 teaspoon vanilla extract.

Directions:

Add all ingredients to a blender and blend until completely smooth.
Adjust sweetness with erythritol if desired.
Pour into a glass.
Serve and enjoy your smoothie!

Variations:

Use coconut milk instead of almond milk.
Add a scoop of chocolate keto protein powder.
Mix in a tablespoon of almond or peanut butter.

Tips:

Use frozen avocado for a thicker, frostier texture.
Add a pinch of cayenne pepper for a chocolate kick.

Nutrition Information (per serving):

Calories 470, Protein 11g, Total Carbs 20g, Fiber 13g, 7g, Fat 41g, Cholesterol 0mg, Sodium 90mg, Potassium 520mg.

Recipe 26: Matcha Smoothie

Prep. time: 4min | Cook time: 10 min | Serves: 2

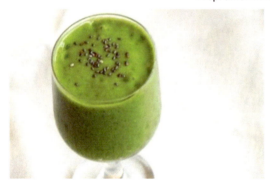

Ingredients:

1 cup unsweetened almond milk
1/2 avocado
2 tablespoons unsweetened cocoa powder
2 tablespoons almond butter
1 tablespoon chia seeds
1 tablespoon erythritol (optional)
1/2 teaspoon vanilla extract.

Directions:

Add all ingredients to a blender and blend until completely smooth.
Adjust sweetness with erythritol if desired.
Pour into a glass.
Serve and enjoy your smoothie!

Variations:

Use almond milk instead of coconut milk.
Substitute cashew butter for almond butter.
Add a handful of fresh spinach or kale.

Tips:

Use culinary matcha powder for a vibrant green color.
Add a squeeze of lemon or lime juice for extra brightness.

Nutrition (per serving):

Calories 38o, Protein 7.4g, Total Carbs 11g, Fiber 8g, 3g, Fat 37g, Cholesterol 0mg, Sodium 75mg, Potassium 460mg.

Recipe 27: Vanilla Smoothie

Prep. time: 5 min | Cook time: 10 min | Serves: 1-2

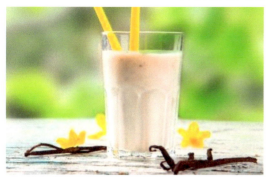

Directions:

Add all ingredients to a blender and blend until completely smooth.
Pour into a glass.
Serve and enjoy your smoothie!

Nutrition Information (per serving):

Calories 365, Protein 5.3g, Total Carbs 10.4g, Fiber 7.1g, 3g, Fat 13g, Cholesterol 0mg, Sodium 45mg, Potassium 256mg.

Ingredients:

1 cup unsweetened almond milk
1/2 cup full-fat cottage cheese
2 tablespoons almond butter
1 tablespoon chia seeds
1 tablespoon erythritol
1 teaspoon vanilla extract.

Recipe 28: Strawberry Smoothie

Prep. time: 5 min | Cook time: 10 min | Serves: 1-2

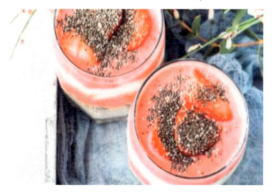

Directions:

Add all ingredients to a blender and blend
Adjust sweetness with erythritol if favored.
Pour into a glass
Serve and enjoy your smoothie!

Variations:

Use coconut milk in place of almond milk.
Add a scoop of strawberry or vanilla keto protein powder.
Mix in a few sparkling mint leaves.

Tips:

Use frozen yogurt in place of Greek yogurt for a thicker texture.
Add a squeeze of lemon juice for extra brightness.

Nutrition (per serving):

Calories 380, Protein 13g, Total Carbs 15g, Fiber 8g, Fat 27g, Cholesterol 10mg, Sodium 190mg, Potassium 350mg.

Ingredients:

1 cup unsweetened almond milk
half cup frozen strawberries
1/4 cup complete-fats Greek yogurt
2 tablespoons almond butter
1 tablespoon chia seeds
1 tablespoon erythritol (non-obligatory)
1/2 teaspoon vanilla extract.

Recipe 29: Coffee Smoothie

Prep. time: 5 min | Cook time: 10 min | Serves: 1-2

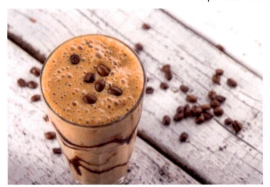

Directions:

Add all ingredients to a blender and mix very well.
Adjust sweetness with erythritol if desired.
Pour into a glass, then serve and enjoy your smoothie!

Nutrition Information (per serving):

Calories 310, Protein 11g, Total Carbs 10g, Fiber 7g, 3g, Fat 25g, Cholesterol 0mg, Sodium 200mg, Potassium 430mg.

Ingredients:

1 cup brewed espresso or bloodless brew, chilled
1/2 cup unsweetened almond milk
2 tablespoons almond butter
1 tablespoon chia seeds
1 tablespoon erythritol (optional)
1 teaspoon vanilla extract
1/four teaspoon cinnamon.

Recipe 30: Raspberry Lemon Smoothie

Prep. time: 5 min | Cook time: 5 min | Serves: 2

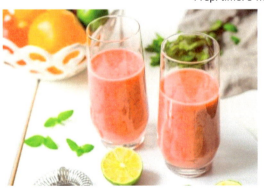

Directions:

Add all ingredients to a blender and mix till smooth.
Adjust sweetness with erythritol if favored.
Pour into a glass and enjoy!

Nutrition Information (per serving):

Calories 380, Protein 13g, Total Carbs 15g, Fiber 8g, Fat 27g, Cholesterol 10mg, Sodium 190mg, Potassium 350mg.

Ingredients:

1 cup unsweetened almond milk
half cup frozen raspberries
1/four cup full-fat Greek yogurt
2 tablespoons almond butter
1 tablespoon chia seeds
1 tablespoon lemon juice
1 tablespoon erythritol (optional).

CHAPTER 3: NUTRITIOUS SNACKS AND LIGHT BITES

3.1. EASY AND TASTY SNACK IDEAS

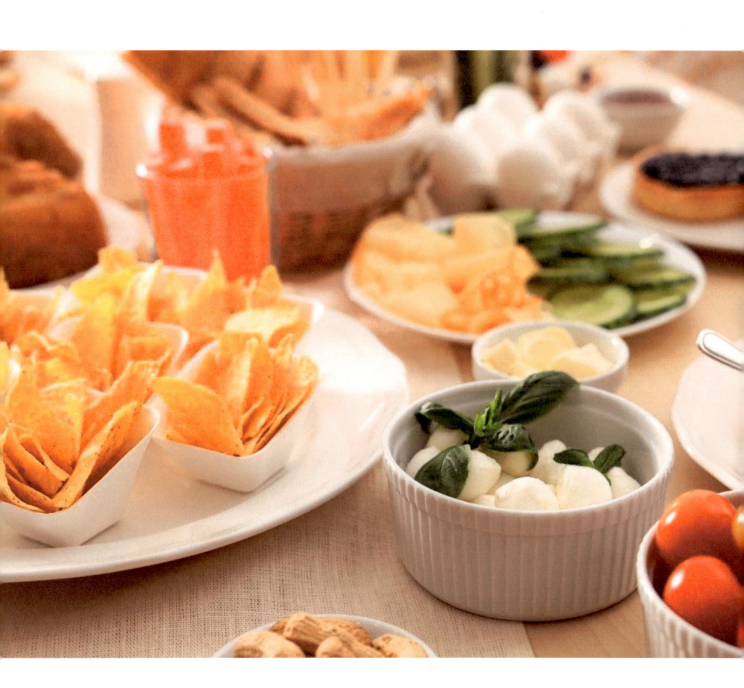

Recipe 31: Edamame with Twist

Prep. time: 10min | Cook time: 5-7 min | Serves: 3

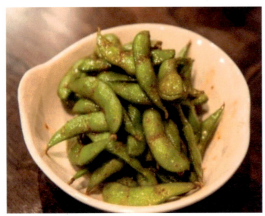

Ingredients:

1 cup frozen shelled edamame
1 tablespoon olive oil
½ teaspoon garlic powder
¼ teaspoon smoked paprika
1 Pinch of purple pepper flakes (optional)
1 pinch of sea salt.

Directions:

Thaw the frozen edamame and the rest of the ingredients in order. Pat dry with a paper towel.
Heat olive oil in a pan over medium heat
Add the edamame, garlic powder, smoked paprika, and red pepper flakes (if using).
Sauté for 5-7 minutes, stirring occasionally, until Edamame is heated through and barely blistered.
Sprinkle with sea salt to flavor
Serve and enjoy!

Variations:

Add a sprinkle of dietary yeast for a cheesy taste.
Drizzle with low-sodium soy sauce or tamari for a savory twist.

Nutrition Information:

Calories: 180, Protein: 12g, Carbohydrates: 10g, Fat: 8g, Fiber: 5g, Cholesterol: 0mg, Sodium: 50mg, Potassium: 200mg.

Recipe 32: Roasted Chickpeas with Herbs

Prep. time: 10 min | Cook time: 25 min | Serves: 2-4

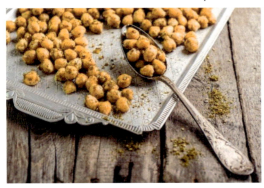

Ingredients:

1 can (15 oz) chickpeas, drained and rinsed
1 tablespoon olive oil
1/2 teaspoon dried oregano
1/4 teaspoon garlic powder
1/4 teaspoon ground cumin
1 Pinch of black pepper
Sea salt to taste.

Directions:

Preheat oven to 400°F (200°C). Line a baking sheet with parchment paper.
Pat the chickpeas dry with a paper towel.
Toss the chickpeas with olive oil, oregano, garlic powder, cumin, and black pepper in a bowl.
Spread the chickpeas on the prepared baking sheet in a single layer.
Roast for 20-25 minutes or until golden brown and crispy.
Sprinkle with sea salt to taste and enjoy!

Nutrition Information:

Calories: 200, Protein: 8g, Carbohydrates: 20g, Fat: 6g, Fiber: 5g, Cholesterol: 0mg, Sodium: 70mg, Potassium: 250mg.

Recipe 33: Roasted Radishes

Prep. time: 10min | Cook time: 25 min | Serves: 3

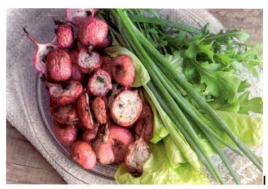

ngredients:

1 bunch of radishes
1 tablespoon olive oil
½ teaspoon dried thyme
1/4 teaspoon garlic powder
Pinch of sea salt
Freshly ground black pepper, to taste.

Directions:

Preheat your oven to 400°F (200°C). Line a baking sheet with parchment paper. Toss the radishes with olive oil, thyme, garlic powder, salt, and pepper. Spread radishes in an unmarried layer on the prepared baking sheet. Roast for 20-25 minutes or until barely browned, flipping halfway.
Serve and enjoy your snack!

Variations:

Add a drizzle of balsamic vinegar for a tangy twist.
Toss in a sprinkle of chopped fresh herbs like rosemary or parsley before serving.

Nutrition Information:

Calories: 30, Protein: 1g, Carbohydrates: 6g, Fat: 1g, Fiber: 2g, Cholesterol: 0mg, Sodium: 300mg, Potassium: 150mg.

Recipe 34: Lentil Patties

Prep. time: 10 min | Cook time: 10 min | Serves: 4

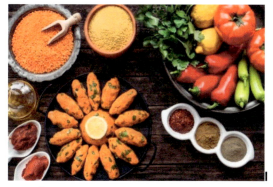

ngredients:

1 cup cooked brown lentils
1 medium sweet potato, roasted and mashed
1/4 cup chopped red onion
1/4 cup chopped fresh cilantro
1 tablespoon whole wheat flour
1/2 teaspoon ground cumin
1/4 teaspoon chili powder
Sea salt and black pepper, to taste
Olive oil for cooking.

Directions:

Mash together the cooked lentils and roasted sweet potato in a large bowl.
Stir in red onion, cilantro, flour, cumin, chili powder, salt, and pepper.
Form the mixture into 4-6 patties. Heat olive oil in a skillet over medium heat.
Cook the patties for 3-4 minutes per side or until golden brown and heated through. Serve warm with your favorite sauce.

Variations:

For extra vegetables, add grated carrots or shredded zucchini. Instead of lentils, use a different type of bean, such as chickpeas or black beans.

Nutrition Information (per serving):

Calories: 280, Protein: 12g, Carbohydrates: 40g, Fat: 8g, Fiber: 10g, Cholesterol: 0mg, Sodium: 98(depending on salt added), Potassium: 450mg.

Recipe 35: Quinoa And Veggie Stuffed Mushrooms

Prep. time: 10 min | Cook time: 15 min | Serves: 2

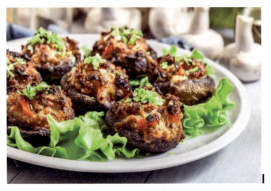

ngredients:

4 large portobello mushrooms
1 cup cooked quinoa
1/2 cup chopped vegetables (such as bell pepper, zucchini, spinach)
1/4 cup chopped red onion
1 clove garlic, minced
1/4 cup crumbled feta cheese
1 tablespoon chopped fresh parsley
1/4 teaspoon dried oregano
2 tablespoons of olive oil for cooking
Sea salt and black pepper, to taste.

Directions:

Preheat the oven to 400°F (200°C). Line a baking sheet with parchment paper. Brush the tops of the portobello mushrooms with olive oil. Season with salt and pepper. Place the mushrooms with the side down on the prepared baking sheet. Bake for 10 minutes.

Meanwhile, heat olive oil in a skillet over medium heat. Sauté onion and garlic until softened.

Add chopped vegetables and cook until tender-crisp.

Stir in cooked quinoa, feta cheese (if using), parsley, and oregano season with salt and pepper.

Remove the mushrooms from the oven and fill the caps with the quinoa mixture.

Bake for an additional 10-15 minutes or until heated through. Serve hot.

Nutritional Information (per serving):

Calories: 280, Protein: 12g, Carbohydrates: 40g, Fat: 8g, Fiber: 10g, Cholesterol: 0mg, Sodium: 98(depending on salt added), Potassium: 450mg.

Recipe 36: Baked Eggplant Fries

Prep. time: 10 min | Cook time: 20-25 min | Serves: 3

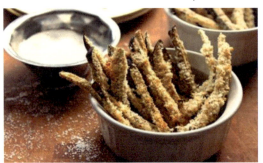

Ingredients:

1 medium eggplant, sliced into sticks
1/four cup breadcrumbs
1/four cup grated Parmesan cheese
1/four cup of panko breadcrumbs
1 tablespoon of olive oil
½ teaspoon dried oregano
1 Pinch of garlic powder
Sea salt and black pepper, to taste.

Directions:

Preheat your oven to 400°F (200°C). Line a baking sheet with parchment paper. In a shallow bowl, combine breadcrumbs, Parmesan cheese (if used), panko breadcrumbs, oregano, garlic powder, salt, and pepper. Arrange the eggplant slices on a plate. Lightly coat every slice with olive oil.

Dredge the oiled eggplant slices within the breadcrumb mixture, coating lightly. Place the breaded eggplant slices in a single layer on the prepared baking sheet.

Bake for 20-25 minutes or until golden brown and soft, flipping midway through.

Serve warm with your favorite dipping sauce, like marinara or ranch dressing.

Nutritional Information (according to serving):

Calories: 400, Protein: 15g, Carbohydrates: 40g, Fat: 18g, Fiber: 5g, Cholesterol: 10mg, Sodium 130, Potassium: 420mg.

Recipe 37: Baked Pears With Walnuts

Prep. time: 10 min | Cook time: 25 min | Serves: 2-3

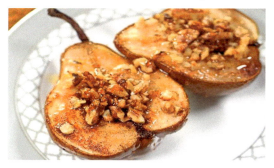

Ingredients:

2 ripe pears, halved and cored
1/four cup chopped walnuts
1 tablespoon maple syrup or dates
1/2 teaspoon ground cinnamon
Pinch of ground nutmeg
1 tablespoon crumbled goat cheese
(optional).

Directions:

Preheat oven to 375°F (190°C). Line a baking dish with parchment paper. Place the pear halves, reduced aspect down, inside the baking dish. Add chopped walnuts, maple syrup or dates, cinnamon, and nutmeg in a small bowl. Spoon the walnut mixture calmly over the cut aspects of the pears. Bake for 20-25 minutes or till the pears are tender and barely golden brown. Top with crumbled goat cheese (optionally available) and serve hot

Variations:

For a tangy twist, drizzle the pears with balsamic vinegar before baking. Substitute chopped pecans or almonds for the walnuts.

Nutritional Information:

Calories: 280, Protein: 2g, Carbohydrates: 60g, Fat: 8g, Fiber: 6g, Cholesterol: 0mg, Sodium 190mg, Potassium: 290mg.

Recipe 38: Cauliflower Fritters

Prep. time: 20 min | Cook time: 15 min | Serves: 4

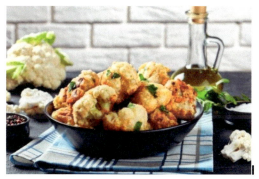

ngredients:

1 large head of cauliflower
1 cup all-purpose flour
1/2 cup grated Parmesan cheese
1/2 cup finely chopped fresh parsley
2 large eggs
1/2 cup milk
1 tsp baking powder
1 tsp salt
1/2 tsp black pepper
1/4 tsp garlic powder
1/4 tsp onion powder
Vegetable oil for frying.

Directions:

Remove the leaves and core from the cauliflower. Cut into florets and steam or boil until tender but not mushy (5-7 minutes). Drain and cool slightly. To make the Batter, Whisk together the flour, Parmesan, parsley, baking powder, salt, pepper, garlic powder, and onion powder. Beat eggs and mix in milk. Add to dry ingredients and stir until combined. Fold cooked cauliflower florets into the batter until well-coated.

Heat 1/2 inch of oil in a skillet over medium-high heat. Drop a spoonful of batter into the hot oil.

Fry in batches, 2-3 minutes per side, until golden brown and crispy. Drain on paper towels.

Serve hot, garnished with parsley. Pair with aioli, ranch, or marinara sauce.

Nutritional Information (per serving):

Calories: 320, Protein: 12g, Carbohydrates: 35g, Fiber: 5g, Sugars: 4g, Fat: 16g, Saturated Fat: 4g, Cholesterol: 85mg, Sodium: 780mg.

Recipe 39: Baked Zucchini Patties

Prep. time: 20 min | Cook time: 25 min | Serves: 4

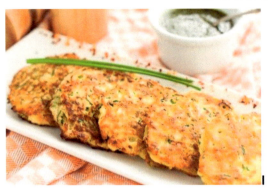

ngredients:

2 medium zucchinis
1 large egg
1/2 cup wheat breadcrumbs
1/4 cup parmesan
2 tablespoons fresh basil, chopped
1 clove garlic, crushed into
Pinch of salt
1/4 teaspoon black pepper
Cooking spray.

Directions:

Preheat the oven to 200°C. Line a baking sheet with parchment paper. Combine the grated zucchini, egg, breadcrumbs, Parmesan cheese, basil, garlic, salt, and black pepper in a large bowl. Stir well until everything is incorporated.

Shape approximately 1/4 cup of zucchini mixture into a patty. Place the patties on the prepared baking sheet, then lightly spritz them with cooking spray.

Bake for about 20-25 minutes or until golden and crispy; they turn over halfway through the cooking time. Serve and enjoy your patties.

Nutrition Information (per serving of 2 patties):

Calories: 140, Protein: 8g, Carbs: 14g, Fiber: 3g, Fat: 5g, Cholesterol: 60mg, Sodium: 320mg, Potassium: 350mg.

Recipe 40: Stuffed Figs Pockets

Prep. time: 10min | Cook time: 25 min | Serves: 4

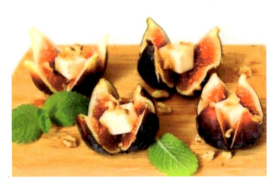

Ingredients:

½ pound of figs
1/2 cup chopped walnuts
1/4 cup chopped pitted dates
1 tablespoon crumbled goat cheese (Optional)
1 tablespoon fresh rosemary, chopped (or 1/2 teaspoon dried)
1 tablespoon olive oil
1/4 cup balsamic vinegar
1 tablespoon honey
1 Pinch of ground black pepper
Fresh rosemary sprig.

Directions:

Preheat oven to 375°F (190°C) and line a baking sheet with parchment paper.

Cut a small incision on top of each fig to create a pocket. In a bowl, mix chopped walnuts, dates, goat cheese (if used), and chopped rosemary. Stuff the figs with this mixture and drizzle with olive oil. Arrange on the baking sheet.

Bake for 15-20 minutes, until figs are softened and filling is warm.

For the balsamic glaze, simmer balsamic vinegar and honey in a small saucepan over medium heat for 5-7 minutes until thickened.

Drizzle the baked figs with the glaze, sprinkle with black pepper, garnish with rosemary, and serve warm or at room temperature. Garnish with a sparkling rosemary sprig and serve warm or at room temperature.

Nutritional Information (according to serving):

Calories: 340, Protein: 4g, Carbohydrates: 16g, Fat:11g, Fiber: 6.7g, Cholesterol: 0mg, Sodium 140, Potassium: 390mg.

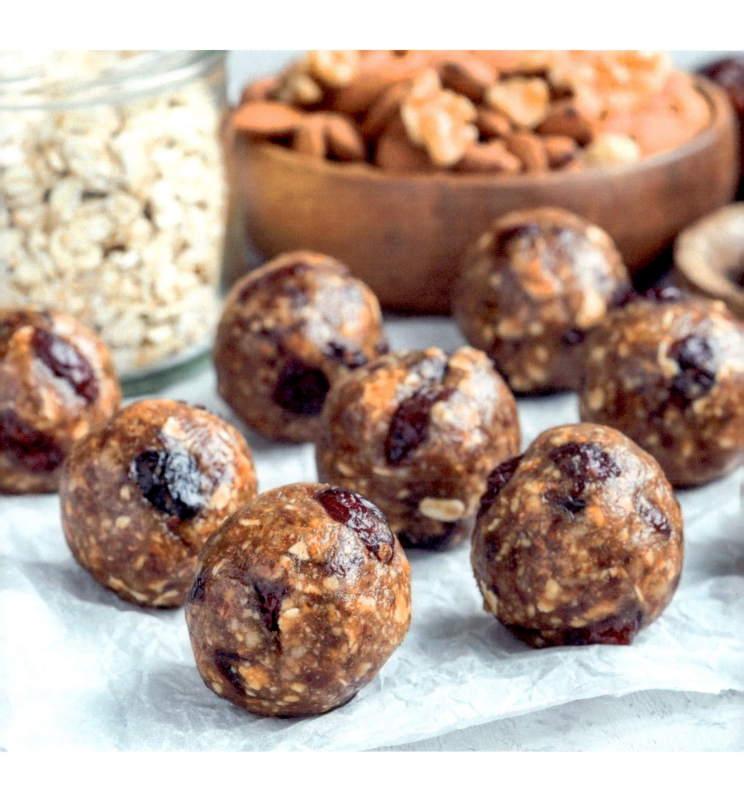

Recipe 41: Oatmeal Almond Bars

Prep. time: 10 min | Cook time: 10 min | Serves: 5

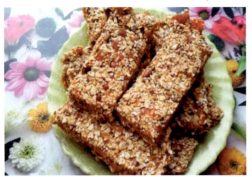

Ingredients:

1 cup rolled oats
half of a cup of creamy almond butter
1/4 cup maple syrup or dates
1/four cup chopped almonds
1/four cup dried cranberries.

Directions:

Mix rolled oats, almond butter, maple syrup, or dates in a large bowl until a thick paste forms. Stir in chopped almonds and dried cranberries.

You can use peanut or cashew butter instead of almond butter and substitute dried cranberries with raisins, dates, or dried cherries. Add chia or flaxseeds for extra fiber. If the mixture is too dry, add a tablespoon of olive oil.

Press the mixture firmly into a baking dish and cut into bars.

Serve and enjoy your bars!

Nutritional Information (per bar):

Calories: 250, Protein: 5g, Carbohydrates: 35g, fiber: 5g, Fat: 10g, Cholesterol: 30mg, Sodium: 80mg (depending on almond butter), Potassium: 200mg.

Recipe 42: Pumpkin Bars

Prep. time: 9 min | Cook time: 20 min | Serves: 5

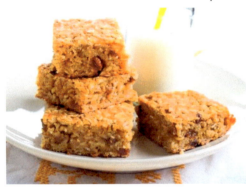

Ingredients:

1 cup rolled oats
1/2 cup canned pumpkin puree
1/4 cup maple syrup
1 teaspoon pumpkin pie spice
1/four cup chopped walnuts.

Directions:

Preheat oven to 350°F (175°C).

Line an 8x8-inch baking dish with parchment paper.

Mix the rolled oats, pumpkin puree, maple syrup, and pumpkin pie spice in a large bowl.

Mix your ingredients very well. Fold in the chopped walnuts. Use pumpkin pie filling rather than pumpkin puree, but lessen the maple syrup to 1/3 cup as the filling is already sweetened.

Add a handful of chocolate chips for a decadent twist.

Press the mixture firmly into the baking dish to make sure the bars maintain their form.

Serve and enjoy your bars

Variation:

Substitute chopped walnuts with different nuts like pecans or almonds.

Tips: Use natural pumpkin puree for a healthier choice.

If the mixture feels too wet, upload a tablespoon of rolled oats.

Nutritional Information (per bar):

Calories: 36.5, Protein: 1.26 grams, Fat: 0.9 grams, Carbohydrates: 6.36 grams, Fiber: 0.95 grams, Cholesterol: 0 mg, Sodium: 0 mg, Potassium: 0 mg.

Recipe 43: Blueberry Almond Bars

Prep. time: 12 min | Cook time: 15 min | Serves: 4-6

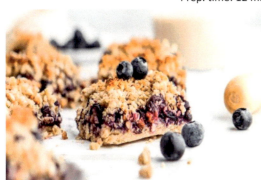

Ingredients:

1 cup rolled oats
1/2 cup creamy almond butter
1/4 cup maple syrup
1/four cup dried blueberries
1/4 cup chopped almonds.

Directions:

Combine rolled oats, almond butter, and maple syrup in a large bowl.
Mix your ingredients until you get a thick paste.
Stir in dried blueberries and chopped almonds.
Press the mixture firmly into the baking dish to keep the bars in shape.
Cut your bars, then serve and enjoy your bars!

Variations:

Substitute different nut butter like peanut butter or cashew butter for almond butter.
You can replace dried blueberries with chopped cherries, dates, or another dried culmination.
Add a pinch of lemon zest for a brighter taste.

Tips: If the combination feels too dry, add a tablespoon of olive oil.

Nutritional Information (per bar):

Calories: 220, Protein: 4g, Carbohydrates: 40g, fiber: 5g, Fat: 8g, Sodium: 40mg, Potassium: 200mg.

Recipe 44: Oatmeal Almond Vanilla Bars

Prep. time: 10 min | Cook time: 25 min | Serves: 5

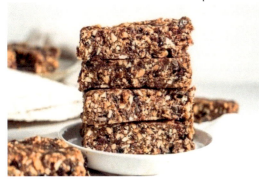

Ingredients:

1 cup rolled oats
1/2 cup mashed ripe banana (about one medium banana)
1/four cup chopped walnuts
1/4 cup maple syrup
1 teaspoon vanilla extract.

Directions:

Preheat oven to 350°F (175°C). Line an 8x8-inch baking dish with parchment paper.
Mix rolled oats, mashed banana, maple syrup, and vanilla extract in a large bowl. Fold in chopped walnuts. Spread evenly into the baking dish.
Bake for 20-25 minutes until golden brown. Allow to cool completely before cutting. Serve and enjoy!

Variations:

Use pecans, almonds, or peanuts instead of walnuts.
Add 1/2 tsp of cinnamon or nutmeg.
Mix in 1/4 cup of dried fruits like raisins or cranberries.

Tips: Let the bars cool completely before cutting. Store in a container for up to three days.

Nutritional Information (per bar):

Calories: 150, Protein: 3g, Carbs: 23g, Fiber: 2g, Fat: 6g, Cholesterol: 25mg, Sodium: 10mg, Potassium: 220mg.

Recipe 45: Chocolate Healthy Bars

Prep. time: 10min | Cook time: 15min | Serves: 5

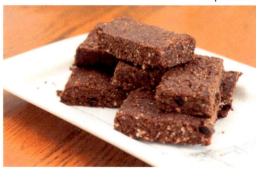

Directions:

Mix the rolled oats, peanut butter, and maple syrup in a large bowl.
Mix very well until you get a thick paste
Stir in the chocolate chips.
Press the mixture firmly right into a baking dish.
Refrigerate until the bars are set, about 2 hours.
Serve and enjoy your bars

Ingredients:

1 cup rolled oats
1/2 cup vegan peanut butter
1/4 cup maple syrup
1/four cup dark chocolate chips

Tips:

Add a tablespoon of almond milk or olive oil if the mixture feels too dry.

Nutritional Information (per bar):

Calories: 260, Protein: 6g, Carbohydrates: 35g, fiber: 5g, Fat: 12g, Cholesterol: 10mg Sodium: 120mg, Potassium: 200mg

Recipe 46: Carrot Healthy Bars

Prep. time: 12 min | Cook time: 15 min | Serves: 5

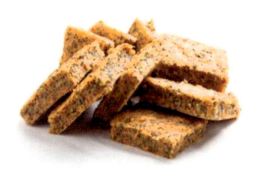

Directions:

Combine rolled oats, grated carrots, maple syrup, cinnamon, and nutmeg in a large bowl and mix very well.
Fold in chopped walnuts.
Press the mixture into an 8x8-inch baking dish covered with parchment paper.
Refrigerate until company, approximately 2 hours.
Cut into bars and serve.

Nutritional Information (per bar):

Calories: 230, Protein: 4g, Carbohydrates: 24g, fiber: 4g, Fat: 8g, Cholesterol: 10mg, Sodium: 40mg, Potassium: 288mg.

Ingredients:

1 cup rolled oats
½ cup grated carrots
1/4 cup chopped walnuts
1/four cup maple syrup
1 teaspoon floor cinnamon
1/4 teaspoon ground nutmeg.

Recipe 47: Cranberry Orange Bars

Prep. time: 10 min | Cook time: 20 min | Serves: 4-6

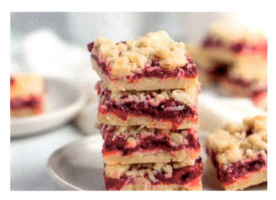

Ingredients:

1 cup rolled oats
½ cup dried cranberries
1/4 cup orange zest
¼ cup maple syrup
½ cup almond butter.

Directions:

Integrate rolled oats, dried cranberries, orange zest, and maple syrup in a vast bowl.
Mix your ingredients very well.
Stir in almond butter until nicely incorporated.
Use a touch of orange juice instead of orange zest for a more intense orange flavor.
Drizzle the bars with melted chocolate
Cut the bars, then serve and enjoy them!

Variations:

You can use other dried results like chopped cherries

Tips:

Chop the dried cranberries into smaller pieces to save them from tearing the bars.
Add a tablespoon or olive oil if the combination feels too dry.

Nutritional Information (per bar):

Calories: 250, Protein: 5g, Carbohydrates: 40g, 3.4g, Fat: 10g, Cholesterol: 15mg, Sodium: 80mg, Potassium: 220mg.

Recipe 48: Rolled Oats Flaxseed bars

Prep. time: 10 min | Cook time: 20 min | Serves: 4-5

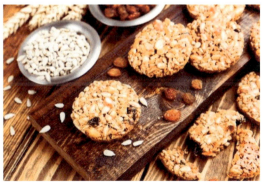

Ingredients:

1 cup rolled oats
1/3 cup natural peanut butter
1/4 cup maple syrup or dates
1/4 cup dark chocolate chips
2 tablespoons ground flaxseeds.

Directions:

Combine the rolled oats, peanut butter, maple syrup or dates, and flaxseeds in a large bowl. Mix properly until the mixture is sticky.
Stir in the chocolate chips.
If the mixture feels too dry, add a tablespoon of olive oil
Roll the mixture into balls
Serve and enjoy your energy balls!

Nutritional Information (per bar):

Calories: 200, Protein: 5g, Carbohydrates: 25g, fiber: 3, Fat: 10g, Cholesterol: 46mg, Sodium: 70mg, Potassium: 150mg.

Recipe 49: Blueberry Bars

Prep. time: 15 min | Cook time: 20 min | Serves: 4-5

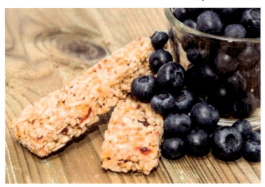

Ingredients:

1 cup rolled oats
half of a cup of creamy almond butter
1/four cup maple syrup or dates
1/four cup dried blueberries
1/four cup chopped almonds.

Directions:

Mix rolled oats, almond butter, maple syrup or dates in a large bowl until a thick paste forms. Stir in dried blueberries and chopped almonds. Press the mixture firmly into an 8x8-inch baking dish lined with parchment paper. Refrigerate for about 2 hours until set. Cut into bars, serve, and enjoy!

Variations:

Use peanut or cashew butter instead of almond butter.

Replace dried blueberries with cherries, dates, or other dried fruits.
Add a pinch of lemon zest for a brighter taste.

Tips:

If it is too dry, add a tablespoon of olive oil.

Press the mixture firmly to ensure the bars hold their shape.

Nutritional Information (per bar):

Calories: 240, Protein: 5g, Carbohydrates: 35g, fiber: 3.5g, Fat: 10g, Cholesterol: 0mg, Sodium: 80mg, Potassium: 210mg.

Recipe 50: Lemon Blueberry Cheesecake

Prep. time: 10 min | Cook time: 25-30min | Serves: 5

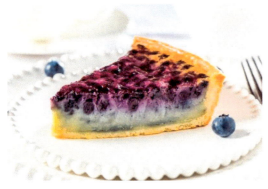

Ingredients:

1 1/2 cups almond flour
1/4 cup melted avocado oil
16 oz cream cheese, softened
1/2 cup powdered erythritol
Two large eggs
1/4 cup lemon juice
1 teaspoon lemon zest
1 cup fresh blueberry.

Directions:

Preheat oven to 350°F (175°C).
Mix the almond flour and avocado oil. Press into a lined 9x9-inch pan. Bake for about 10 minutes.
Beat cream cheese and erythritol until smooth. Beat in eggs, lemon juice, and zest.
Pour into crust; sprinkle the top with blueberries.
Bake for 25-30 minutes until set.
Cool completely and refrigerate for at least 2 hours before cutting.
Serve and enjoy your Cheesecake.

Nutrition Information (per bar, 16 bars total):

Calories: 180, Protein: 5g, Total Carbs: 6g, Fiber: 1g, Fat: 16g, Sodium: 95mg, Potassium: 90mg.

Recipe 51: Apricot Almond Bars

Prep. time: 10 min | Cook time: 25-30min | Serves: 5

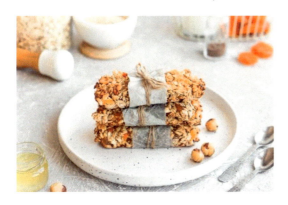

Ingredients:

1 cup dried apricots
 1 cup raw, unsalted almonds
1/2 cup of rolled oats
2 tablespoons ground flaxseed
1 teaspoon vanilla extract
 1/4 tablespoons of water.

Directions:

Pulse the almonds in a food processor until they become very fine.
Stir in the apricots to the desired consistency.
Add rolled oats, flaxseed, vanilla, and cinnamon; process very well to combine.
Add in the water and process until the mixture forms.
Press your mixture into an 8x8-inch pan that is lined with parchment paper
Refrigerate for about 1 hour, then cut into 12 bars.
Serve and enjoy your bars!

Nutrition Information (per bar, 12 bars total):

Calories: 130, Protein: 4g, Total Carbs: 15g, Fiber: 3g, Fat: 7g, Sodium: 1mg, Potassium: 240mg.

CHAPTER 4: SALADS AND SOUPS

4.1.SALADS FULL OF ANTIOXIDANTS

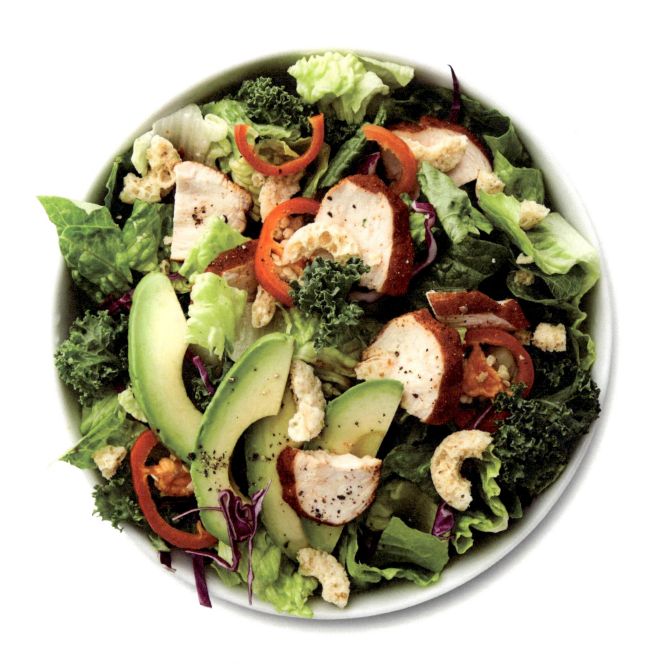

Recipe 52: Classic Caesar Salad

Prep. time: 15 min | Cook time: 25 min | Serves: 4

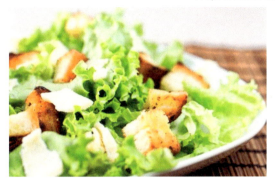

Ingredients:

1 massive head of romaine lettuce, washed and chopped 2 tablespoons grated Parmesan cheese 1/4 cup entire-grain croutons
2 anchovy fillets
For the Dressing:
1/4 cup low-fat plain Greek yogurt
2 tablespoons lemon juice
1 teaspoon Dijon mustard
1 garlic clove, minced
1 tablespoon olive oil
Salt and pepper to taste.

Directions:

Combine the chopped romaine lettuce, Parmesan cheese, and croutons (if using) in a large salad bowl.
Whisk together all the dressing elements in a small bowl until well blended.
Pour the dressing over the salad and toss gently to coat the lettuce leaves.
If using anchovy fillets, place them on top of the salad.
Serve at once.
Massage the dressing into the lettuce leaves for better taste distribution.
Serve and enjoy!

Nutritional Information:

Calories: 130, Protein: 6g, Carbohydrates: 10g, Fiber: 3g, Fat: 8g, Cholesterol: 5mg, Sodium: 280mg, Potassium: 380mg

Recipe 53: Southwestern Black Bean Salad

Prep. time: 15 min | Cook time: 20 min | Serves: 4

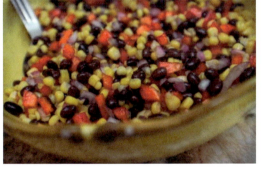

Ingredients:

1 (15 oz) can black beans, rinsed and drained
1 cup corn kernels (fresh or frozen)
1 red bell pepper, diced
1/2 red onion, diced
1/4 cup chopped fresh cilantro
1 avocado, diced
For the Dressing:
2 tablespoons lime juice
2 tablespoons olive oil
1 teaspoon ground cumin
1 teaspoon chili powder
Salt and pepper to taste.

Directions:

Combine the black beans, corn, bell pepper, red onion, cilantro, and diced avocado in a large bowl.
In a small bowl, whisk together the lime juice, olive oil, cumin, chili powder, salt, and pepper.
Pour the dressing over the salad and toss gently to combine.
Refrigerate for at least 30 minutes to allow flavors to blend.
Serve chilled or at room temperature.

Nutritional Information (per serving):

Calories: 220, Protein: 7g, Carbohydrates: 28g, Fiber: 9g, Fat: 10g, Cholesterol: 0mg, Sodium: 120mg, Potassium: 590mg.

Recipe 54: Kale and Blueberry Salad with Avocado and Almonds

Prep. time: 10 min | Cook time: 20 min | Serves: 4

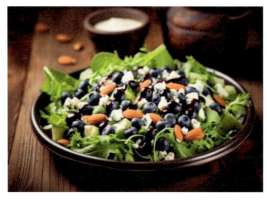

Directions:

Put the chopped kale in a large salad bowl
Add the diced avocado, blueberries, and sliced almonds.
Put in and lightly mix.
Serve it immediately.

Nutritional Information (per serving):

Calories: 201, Protein: 5g, Carbohydrates: 18g, Fiber: 8g, Fat: 9g, Cholesterol: 0mg, Sodium: 130mg, Potassium: 380mg.

Ingredients:

1 large bunch of kale, stems removed
1 Ripe Avocado, medium
1 cup Fresh Blueberries
1/4 cup Slivered almonds.

Recipe 55: Southwestern Black Bean Salad

Prep. time: 15 min | Cook time: 20 min | Serves: 4

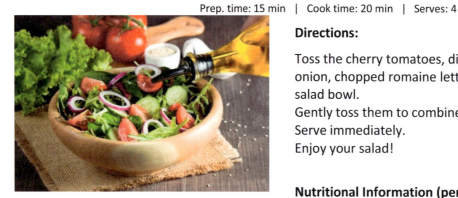

Directions:

Toss the cherry tomatoes, diced cucumber, sliced red onion, chopped romaine lettuce, and parsley in a large salad bowl.
Gently toss them to combine.
Serve immediately.
Enjoy your salad!

Nutritional Information (per serving):

Calories: 40, Total Fat: 0g, Saturated Fat: 0g, Cholesterol: 0mg, Sodium: 20mg, Total Carbohydrates: 8g, Dietary Fiber: 3g, Protein: 2g, Potassium: 460mg.

Ingredients:

1 large head of romaine, washed and chopped
1 cup cherry tomatoes, halved
1 cucumber, small dice
1/2 red onion, thinly sliced
1/4 cup fresh parsley, chopped.

Recipe 56: Citrus Avocado Salad with Pomegranate

Prep. time: 12 min | Cook time: 20 min | Serves: 3-4

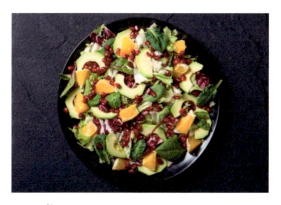

Ingredients:

4 cups mixed salad greens
1 large orange, peeled and segmented
1 grapefruit, peeled and segmented
1 ripe avocado, sliced
1/4 cup pomegranate seeds
2 tablespoons sliced almonds
2 tablespoons extra virgin olive oil
1 tablespoon orange juice
1 teaspoon of honey
1/4 teaspoon of ground cinnamon.

Directions:

Toss the salad greens with the orange segments, grapefruit pieces, avocado slices, pomegranate seeds, and almonds.
Combine olive oil, orange juice, honey, and cinnamon with a whisk.
Drizzle dressing over salad; toss gently to combine.
Serve immediately, and enjoy your salad!

Nutritional Information (per 4 servings):

Calories 200, 3g protein, 18g total carbs, 6g fiber, 15g fat, 10mg sodium, 400mg potassium.

Recipe 57: Anti- Oxidant cabbage salad

Prep. time: 10 min | Cook time: 20 min | Serves: 4

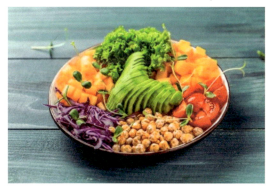

Ingredients:

2 cups chopped red cabbage
1 cup steamed edamame
1 cup cherry tomatoes, halved
1 cup of diced mango
1/4 cup fresh cilantro, chopped
2 tablespoons extra-virgin olive oil
2 tablespoons rice vinegar
1 teaspoon grated ginger
1/4 teaspoon of turmeric
1/8 teaspoon black pepper.

Directions:

Mix the red cabbage, edamame, cherry tomatoes, mango, and cilantro in a big bowl.
Combine the olive oil, rice vinegar, ginger, turmeric, and black pepper in a small bowl; whisk them well.
Pour dressing over the salad and toss to combine.
Divide into bowls and serve.

Nutrition Information (per serving, 4 servings total):

Calories 320, 10g protein, 45g total carbs, 7g fiber, 13g fat, Sodium: 25mg, Potassium: 550mg.

Recipe 58: Cauliflower Tabbouleh

Prep. time: 10 min | Cook time: 20 min | Serves: 3

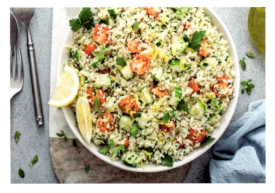

Ingredients:

4 cups cauliflower rice, about 1 medium
head, pulsed in a food processor
1 cup fresh parsley, finely chopped
1/2 cup of fresh mint, minced
1/4 cup red bell pepper, minced
1/4 cup cucumber, finely diced
2 tablespoons fresh lemon juice
2 tablespoons of extra-virgin olive oil
1 clove garlic, minced
1/4 teaspoon cumin,
1/8 teaspoon of black pepper.

Directions:

Combine the large bowl of cauliflower rice, parsley, mint, red
bell pepper, and cucumber.
Whisk together lemon juice, olive oil, crushed garlic, cumin,
and black pepper in a small bowl.
Pour the dressing over the salad and toss.
Serve and enjoy your salad!

Nutrition Information (per serving, 4 servings total):

Calories: 110, Protein: 3g, Total Carbs: 8g, Fiber: 3g, Fat: 8g,
Sodium: 35mg, Potassium: 400mg.

Recipe 59: Avocado Spinach Salad

Prep. time: 8 min | Cook time: 15 min | Serves: 2-4

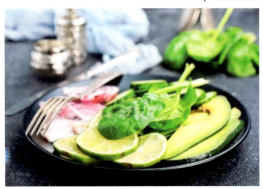

Ingredients:

4 cups fresh baby spinach
1 large avocado, cut into chunks
1/4 cup red onion, cut into very thin dices
2 tablespoons pumpkin seeds
2 tablespoons of extra virgin olive oil
1 tablespoon apple cider vinegar
1 teaspoon Dijon mustard
 1/4 teaspoon of garlic powder
1/8 teaspoon of black pepper.

Directions:

Add spinach to a large bowl, together with the avocado, red
onion, and pumpkin seeds.
In a small bowl, whisk together olive oil, apple cider vinegar,
Dijon mustard, garlic powder, and black pepper.
Drizzle the dressing over the salad and lightly toss it
together.
Serve immediately.

Nutrition Information (per serving, 4 servings total):

Calories: 250, Protein: 5g, Carbohydrates: 35g
Fiber: 5g, Fat: 10g, Cholesterol: 30mg Sodium: 80mg
(depending on almond butter)
Potassium: 200mg

Recipe 60: Zucchini Noodles salad

Prep. time: 7 min | Cook time: 20 min | Serves: 4

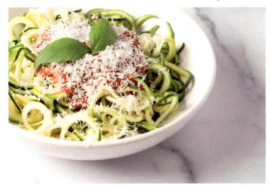

Ingredients:

4 medium zucchinis, spiralized

1/2 cup cherry tomatoes, chopped

1/4 cup pine nuts

1/4 cup chopped fresh basil leaves

2 tablespoons extra-virgin olive oil

2 tablespoons homemade pesto (basil, olive oil, pine nuts, garlic)

1 tablespoon lemon juice

1/4 cup Parmesan cheese, grated (optional)

1/8 teaspoon black pepper.

Directions:

Toss the zucchini noodles with cherry tomatoes, pine nuts, and basil leaves.

Whisk the olive oil, pesto, lemon juice, and black pepper together.

Drizzle the dressing over the salad and toss to coat. If desired, sprinkle Parmesan cheese over the top.

Serve and enjoy your salad.

Nutrition Information (per serving, 4 servings total):

Calories: 200, Protein: 5g, Total Carbs: 7g, Fiber: 2g, Fat: 18g, Sodium: 55mg, Potassium: 450mg.

Recipe 61: Egg and Spinach Salad

Prep. time: 10 min | Cook time: 15 min | Serves: 4

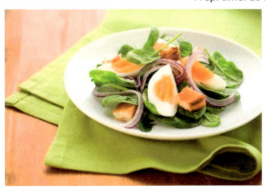

Ingredients:

4 cups of fresh baby spinach

4 big eggs, boiled and quartered

1/4 cup red onion, thinly sliced

1/4 cup sliced almonds

2 tablespoons extra-virgin olive oil

1 Tablespoons of apple cider vinegar

1 teaspoon of Dijon mustard Garlic powder

1/8 teaspoon of black pepper

1 tablespoon fresh chives, chopped.

Directions:

Toss the spinach, quartered eggs, red onions, and slivered almonds into a bowl.

In a small bowl, whisk olive oil, apple cider vinegar, Dijon mustard, garlic powder, and black pepper.

Drizzle dressing over salad and gently toss to combine.

Serve and enjoy your salad!

Nutrition Information (per serving, 4 servings total):

Calories: 190, Protein: 10g, Total Carbs: 4g, Fiber: 2g, Fat: 16g, Sodium: 95mg, Potassium: 400mg.

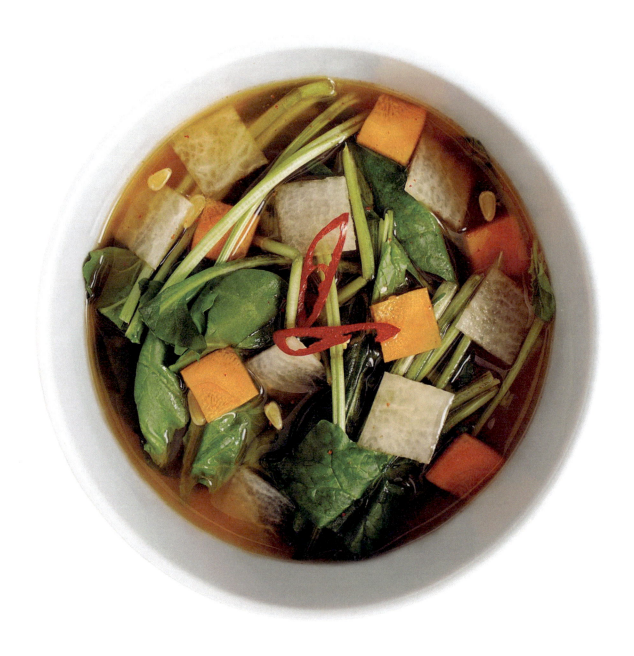

Recipe 62: Butternut Squash Soup

Prep. time: 35 min | Cook time: 30 min | Serves: 4

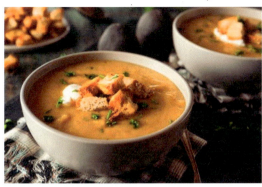

Directions:

Sauté onion and garlic in a pot until it becomes fragrant
Add squash, broth, and thyme; bring to a boil.
Reduce heat and simmer for 20 minutes until squash is tender.
Blend soup until smooth.

Nutritional Information (per serving):

Calories: 120, Protein: 2g, Carbs: 28g, Fiber: 5g, Fat: 1g, Cholesterol: 0mg, Sodium: 140mg, Potassium: 720mg.

Ingredients:

1 butternut squash, peeled and cubed
1 onion, diced
3 garlic cloves, minced
4 cups vegetable broth
1 teaspoon dried thyme
Salt and pepper to taste.

Recipe 63: Lentil Vegetable Soup

Prep. time: 10 min | Cook time: 40 min | Serves: 6

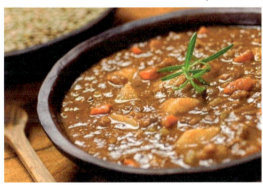

Directions:

Toss the cherry tomatoes, diced cucumber, sliced red onion, chopped romaine lettuce, and parsley in a large salad bowl.
Gently toss them to combine.
Serve immediately.
Enjoy your salad!

Nutritional Information (per serving):

Calories: 170, Protein: 10g, Carbs: 30g, Fiber: 13g, Fat: 1g, Cholesterol: 0mg, Sodium: 120mg, Potassium: 600mg.

Ingredients:

1 cup dried lentils
1 onion, diced
3 carrots, sliced
3 celery stalks, sliced
4 cups vegetable broth
2 teaspoons dried basil
Salt and pepper to taste.

Recipe 64: Tomato Basil Soup

Prep. time: 10min | Cook time: 30 min | Serves: 3-4

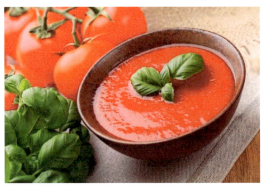

Directions:

Sauté onion and garlic in olive oil in a pot.
Add tomatoes, broth, and basil; simmer for 20 minutes.
Blend or puree soup until smooth.
Season with salt and pepper.
Serve and enjoy your soup!

Nutritional Information (per serving):

Calories: 130, Protein: 3g, Carbs: 15g, Fiber: 4g, Fat: 6g, Cholesterol: 0mg, Sodium: 180mg, Potassium: 680mg.

Ingredients:

1 onion, diced
3 garlic cloves, minced
2 (14.5oz) cans diced tomatoes
2 cups vegetable broth
1/2 cup fresh basil, chopped
2 tablespoons olive oil
Salt and pepper to taste.

Recipe 65: Chicken and Sweet Potato Soup

Prep. time: 10 min | Cook time: 20 min | Serves: 6

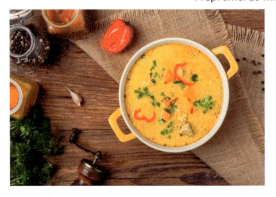

Directions:

Heat the olive oil in a large pot over medium heat.
Stir in the onions and celery, and cook until tender, about 5 minutes. Add the garlic and sauté for a minute. Add the chicken and sauté for 5-7 minutes until the ingredients are no longer pink.
Add sweet potatoes, rosemary, thyme, and broth.
Bring to a boil, then reduce heat and simmer for 15–20 minutes until sweet potatoes are tender.
Stir in kale and cook for 3–4 minutes until it wilts.
Add in the lemon juice and pepper.

Nutrition Information (per serving, 6 servings total):

Calories: 220, Protein: 24g, Total Carbs: 20g, Fiber: 3g, Fat: 5g, Sodium: 140mg, Potassium: 650mg

Ingredients:

1 tablespoon olive oil
1 onion, chopped
2 stalks celery, chopped
2 cloves garlic, minced
1 lb boneless, skinless chicken breast cut into bite-sized pieces
2 sweet potatoes, peeled and cubed
1 teaspoon dried rosemary
1 teaspoon dried thyme
6 cups low-sodium chicken broth
2 cups kale, finely chopped
2 tablespoons of lemon juice
1/4 teaspoon pepper
 2 tablespoons fresh parsley, chopped.

Recipe 66: Split Pea Soup

Prep. time: 10 min | Cook time: 60 min | Serves: 6

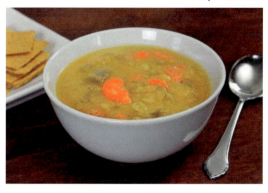

Ingredients:

1 lb dried split peas
1 onion, diced
2 carrots, sliced
2 celery stalks, sliced
6 cups vegetable broth
1 bay leaf
Salt and pepper to taste.

Directions:

Rinse split peas and soak for 1 hour if desired (reduces cooking time).
Sauté onions in a pot until translucent.
Add split peas, carrots, celery, broth, and bay leaf.
Bring to a boil, reduce heat, and simmer for 45-60 minutes.
Remove bay leaf and season with salt and pepper.
Serve and enjoy your soup!

Nutritional Information (per serving):

Calories: 250, Protein: 16g, Carbs: 44g, Fiber: 16g, Fat: 1g, Cholesterol: 0mg, Sodium: 110mg, Potassium: 730mg.

Recipe 67: Roasted Red Pepper and Tomato Soup

Prep. time: 10 min | Cook time: 30 min | Serves: 4

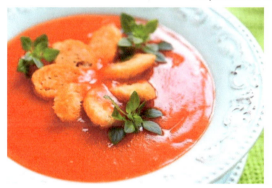

Ingredients:

4 large red bell peppers, halved and seeded
2 lbs ripe tomatoes, halved
1 big onion, quartered
4 garlic cloves
2 tablespoons extra virgin olive oil
1 teaspoon dried thyme
4 cups low-sodium vegetable broth
2 tablespoons balsamic vinegar
1/4 cup fresh basil leaves, torn
1/4 teaspoon. black pepper
2 tablespoons plain Greek yogurt for serving.

Directions:

Preheat the oven to 425°F (220°C).
Lay the bell peppers, tomatoes, onion, and garlic on a large baking sheet.
Drizzle olive oil over the vegetables, and sprinkle thyme over the vegetables.
Bake for 25-30 minutes or until tender vegetables are slightly charred.
Transfer the roasted vegetables to a blender; add the broth and purée until smooth. Pour the soup into a pot and add balsamic vinegar, basil, and pepper.
Serve and enjoy your soup.

Nutrition Information (per serving, 6 servings total):

Calories: 120, Protein: 3g, Total Carbs: 15g, Fiber: 4g, Fat: 6g, Sodium: 70mg, Potassium: 600mg.

Recipe 68: Mushroom and Barley Soup

Prep. time: 12 min | Cook time: 35 min | Serves: 4-6

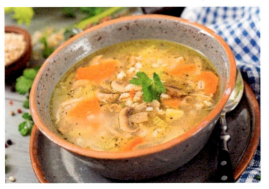

Ingredients:

1 tablespoon olive oil, 1 onion, chopped, 2 carrots, diced, 2 stalks celery, diced, 8 oz mushrooms, sliced, 2 cloves garlic, minced. 1/2 cup pearl barley, rinsed 6 cups vegetable broth, low-sodium 1 teaspoon of dried thyme
1 bay leaf 2 cups chopped kale 2 tablespoons balsamic vinegar and 1/4 teaspoon of black pepper, 2 tablespoons of chopped fresh parsley.

Directions:

Heat olive oil in a large pot over medium heat. Add the onion, carrot, and celery, and cook until the vegetables are soft, about 5 minutes. Add the mushrooms and cook for an additional 5 minutes.
Add the garlic and cook for 1 minute.
Add the barley, broth, thyme, and bay leaf. Bring to a boil, then reduce heat and simmer for 30-35 minutes until barley is tender.
Add the kale and cook for 3-4 minutes until wilted. Remove the bay leaf. Stir in balsamic vinegar and pepper.
Serve and enjoy your soup!

Nutrition Information (per serving):

Calories: 160, Protein: 5g, Total Carbs: 28g, Fiber: 5g, Fat: 4g, Sodium: 110mg, Potassium: 500mg.

Recipe 69: Curried Cauliflower and Lentil Soup

Prep. time: 15 min | Cook time: 25 min | Serves: 4-6

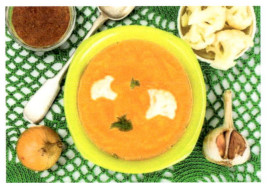

Ingredients:

1 tablespoon olive oil
1 onion, chopped and 2 cloves garlic, minced. 1 tablespoon grated fresh ginger
2 teaspoons curry powder
1 teaspoon turmeric powder
1 head cauliflower, broken into florets
1 cup of rinsed red lentils
6 cups low-sodium vegetable broth
1 (14.5 oz) can no-salt-added diced tomatoes
2 cups baby spinach
2 tablespoons lemon juice
1/4 cup fresh cilantro leaves

Directions:

Drizzle the olive oil into a large pot over medium heat. Add the onion, and cook until the onion is soft, for around 5 minutes.
Add the garlic, ginger, curry powder, and turmeric. Sauté for 1 minute, until fragrant.
Stir in cauliflower, lentils, broth, and tomatoes. Bring to a boil, then reduce heat and simmer for 20-25 minutes or until the cauliflower and lentils are tender.
Add the spinach and cook for two more minutes, until wilted. Stir in lemon juice, cilantro, and pepper.
Serve and enjoy your soup!

Nutrition Information (per serving):

Calories: 190, Protein: 11g, Total Carbs: 30g, Fiber: 8g, Fat: 4g, Sodium: 95mg, Potassium: 650mg.

Recipe 70: White Bean and Kale Soup with Rosemary

Prep. time: 10 min | Cook time: 20 min | Serves: 6

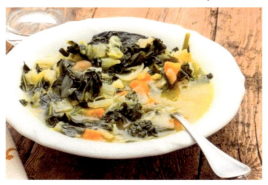

Directions:

In a large pot, heat olive oil over medium heat. Add onion, carrots, and celery. Cook until softened, about 5 minutes. Add the garlic and sauté for a minute.

Stir in the beans, broth, rosemary, and bay leaf, and bring to a boil. Reduce the heat and simmer for at least 15 minutes. Put in the kale and cook for another five minutes until tender. Remove the bay leaf—season with lemon juice and pepper.

Ingredients:

1 tablespoon olive oil, 1 large onion, chopped, 2 carrots, diced, 2 sticks of diced celery, 3 cloves garlic, minced, 2 (15 oz) cans white beans, no-salt-added, drained and rinsed. 6 cups low-sodium vegetable broth. 2 teaspoons fresh rosemary, chopped. 1 bay leaf, 4 cups chopped kale
2 tablespoons lemon juice. 1/4 teaspoon of ground black pepper. 2 tablespoons fresh parsley, chopped.

Nutrition Information (per serving):

Calories: 200, Protein: 12g, Total Carbs: 32g, Fiber: 8g, Fat: 4g, Sodium: 75mg, Potassium: 650mg

Recipe 71: Tuscan-Style Vegetable and Chickpea Soup

Prep. time: 10 min | Cook time: 25 min | Serves: 5

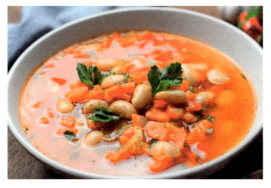

Directions:

In a large pot, heat olive oil over medium heat. Add onion, carrots, and celery. Cook until softened, about 5 minutes. Add garlic and zucchini. Cook for 3 minutes.
Add tomatoes, chickpeas, broth, oregano, and dried basil. Bring to a boil, then reduce heat and simmer for 15 minutes. Add kale and cook for 5 more minutes until tender.
Stir in lemon juice and pepper.
Garnish with fresh basil before serving.
Serve and enjoy your soup!

Ingredients:

1 tablespoon olive oil6 1 onion, diced, 2 carrots, diced, 2 celery stalks, diced
3 garlic cloves, minced,
1 zucchini, diced, 1 (14.5 oz) can no-salt-added diced tomatoes.
1 (15 oz) can no-salt-added chickpeas, drained and rinsed,
6 cups low-sodium vegetable broth,
1 teaspoon dried oregano
1 teaspoon dried basil, 2 cups chopped kale,
2 tablespoons lemon juice, 1/4 teaspoon black pepper, 2 tablespoons fresh basil, chopped.

Nutrition Information (per serving):

Calories: 180, Protein: 8g, Total Carbs: 30g, Fiber: 7g, Fat: 4g, Sodium: 90mg, Potassium: 600mg.

73

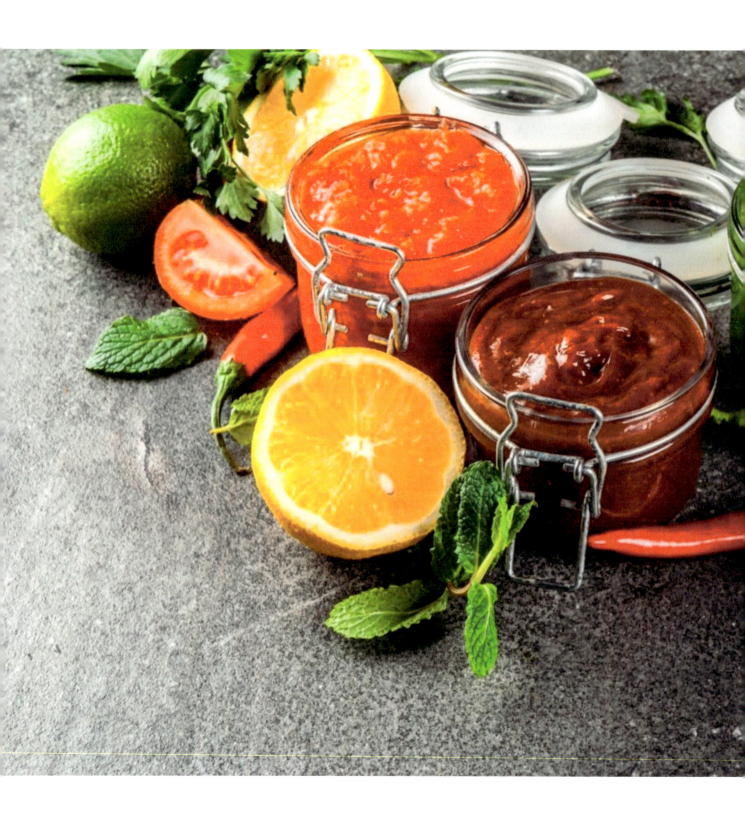

Recipe 72: Balsamic Vinaigrette

Prep. time: 5min | Cook time: 10 min | Serves: 8 (2 tablespoons per serving)

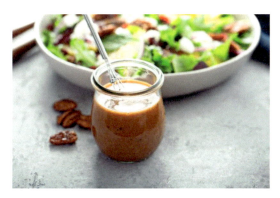

Directions:

Whisk all ingredients together until emulsified.
Use your vinaigrette!

Nutritional Information (per serving):

Calories: 60, Protein: 0g, Carbs: 3g, Fiber: 0g, Fat: 6g,
Cholesterol: 0mg, Sodium: 25mg, Potassium: 30mg.

Ingredients:

1/2 cup balsamic vinegar
1/4 cup olive oil
2 teaspoons Dijon mustard
2 cloves garlic, minced
1 teaspoon honey
Salt and pepper to taste.

Recipe 73: Lemon Tahini Dressing

Prep. time: 5 min | Cook time: 10 min | Serves: 7(2 tablespoons per serving)

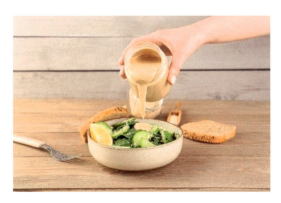

Directions:

Whisk all ingredients together until smooth.
Use your tahini in any salad of your choice!

Nutritional Information (per serving):

Calories: 70, Protein: 2g, Carbs: 3g, Fiber: 1g, Fat: 6g,
Cholesterol: 0mg, Sodium: 25mg, Potassium: 80mg

Ingredients:

1/4 cup tahini
1/4 cup water
2 tablespoons lemon juice
1 garlic clove, minced
Salt and pepper to taste

Recipe 74: Citrus Vinaigrette

Prep. time: 5 min | Cook time: 10 min | Serves: 3

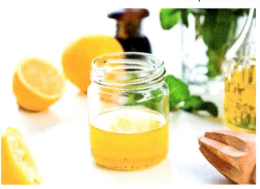

Directions:

Combine all of your ingredients in a jar with a tight-fitting lid.

Shake your ingredients until they are very well combined.

Nutrition Information (per 2 tablespoons serving):

Calories: 85, Fat: 9g, Carbs: 2g, Fiber: 0g, Protein: 0g, Sodium: 25mg, Potassium: 135mg.

Ingredients:

2 tablespoons of orange juice
2 tablespoons of lemon juice
1/4 cup of olive oil
1 teaspoon of Dijon mustard
1/4 teaspoon of dried thyme
1/8 teaspoon of black pepper.

Recipe 75: Raspberry Vinaigrette

Prep. time: 5 min | Cook time: 10 min | Serves: 4

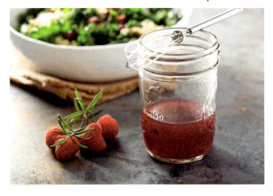

Directions:

Blend all of your ingredients until a smooth consistency is achieved.

You can strain if you wish to remove seeds.

Use and enjoy your vinaigrette!

Nutrition Information (per 2 tablespoons serving):

Calories: 50, Fat: 4g, Carbs: 4g, Fiber: 1g, Protein: 0g, Sodium: 1mg, Potassium: 35mg.

Ingredients:

1/2 cup fresh raspberries
2 tablespoons balsamic vinegar
2 tablespoons olive oil
1 teaspoon honey (optional)
1/4 teaspoon dried thyme
1/8 tsp black pepper.

Recipe 76: Creamy Dill Dressing

Prep. time: 5 min | Cook time: 10 min | Serves: 3

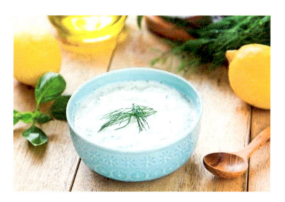

Directions:

Combine the ingredients all together in a bowl.
Use your dressings in salads of your choice!

Nutrition Information (per 2 tablespoons serving):

Calories: 85, Fat: 9g, Carbs: 2g, Fiber: 0g, Protein: 0g, Sodium: 25mg, Potassium: 135mg.

Ingredients:

1/2 cup Greek yogurt
2 tablespoons of fresh dill, chopped
1 tablespoon of lemon juice
1 clove Garlic, minced
1 teaspoon of olive oil
1/8 teaspoon black pepper.

Recipe 77: Asian Sesame Dressing

Prep. time: 5 min | Cook time: 10 min | Serves: 4

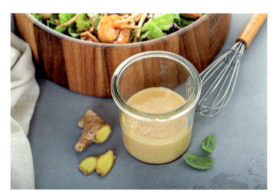

Directions:

Whisk together all ingredients in a small bowl.

Nutrition Information (per 2 tablespoons serving):

Calories: 65, Fat: 7g, Carbs: 1g, Fiber: 0g, Protein: 0g, Sodium: 1mg, Potassium: 15mg.

Ingredients:

2 tablespoons of rice vinegar
1 Tablespoon of sesame oil
1 tablespoon of olive oil
1 teaspoon of grated fresh ginger
1 clove garlic, minced
1 teaspoon of sesame seeds
1/8 teaspoon of ground Black Pepper.

Recipe 78: Lemon Poppy Seed Dressing

Prep. time: 5 min | Cook time: 10 min | Serves: 4

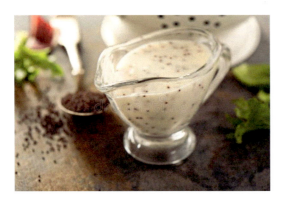

Directions:

Whisk until well combined.

Nutrition Information (per 2 tablespoons serving):

Calories: 80, Fat: 7g, Carbs: 4g, Fiber: 0g, Protein: 0g, Sodium: 1mg, Potassium: 15mg.

Ingredients:

1/4 cup lemon juice
1/4 cup olive oil
1 tablespoon of honey (optional)
1 teaspoon of poppy seeds
1/4 teaspoon of dried mustard
1/8 teaspoon of ground black pepper.

Recipe 79: Maple Balsamic Dressing

Prep. time: 6 min | Cook time: 10 min | Serves: 4-5

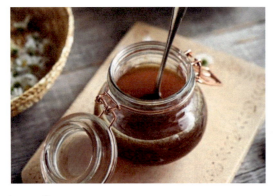

Directions:

Whisk all ingredients together until emulsified.
Use and enjoy your dressing!

Nutrition Information (per 2 tablespoons serving):

Calories: 70, Fat: 6g, Carbs: 5g, Fiber: 0g, Protein: 0g, Sodium: 20mg, Potassium: 30mg.

Ingredients:

3 tablespoons of Balsamic vinegar
2 tablespoons extra virgin olive oil
1 tablespoon of maple syrup
1 teaspoon of Dijon mustard
1/4 teaspoon of garlic powder
1/8 teaspoon of black pepper.

CHAPTER 5: DINNER DELIGHT MAIN COURSES

5.1.FISH AND OMEGA-3 RICH RECIPES

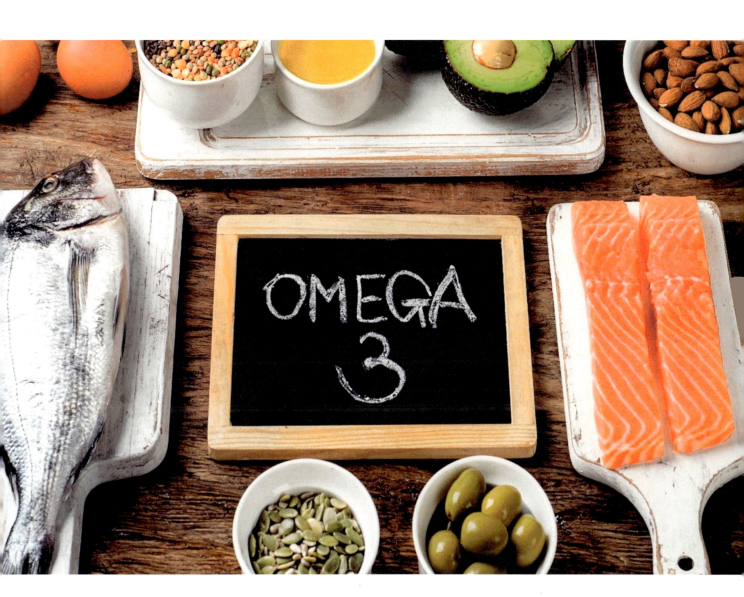

Recipe 80: Baked Salmon with Lemon Dill Sauce

Prep. time: 10 min | Cook time: 20 min | Serves: 4

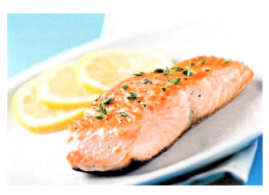

Ingredients:

4 (6 oz) of salmon fillets
1 cup of plain Greek yogurt
2 tablespoons of lemon juice
2 tablespoons of chopped fresh dill
1 garlic clove, minced
Salt and pepper to taste.

Directions:

Preheat your oven to 400°F.
Place the salmon on a baking sheet and season with salt and pepper.
Combine yogurt, lemon juice, dill, and garlic in a small serving bowl for the sauce.
Bake salmon for 12-15 minutes or until opaque in the center.
Serve salmon topped with lemon dill sauce.
Enjoy your dinner!

Nutritional Information (per serving):

Calories: 260, Protein: 34g, Carbs: 4g, Fiber: 0g, Fat: 12g, Cholesterol: 85mg, Sodium: 135mg, potassium: 340mg.

Recipe 81: Cod fillet with tomatoes and olives

Prep. time: 5 min | Cook time: 20 min | Serves: 7

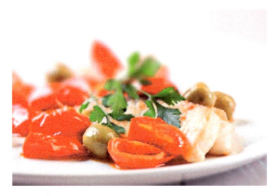

Ingredients:

4 (6 oz) cod fillets
1 (14 oz) can diced tomatoes
1/2 cup pitted kalamata olives
2 tablespoons olive oil
two garlic cloves, minced
1 teaspoon dried oregano
Salt and pepper to taste.

Directions:

Preheat oven to 400°F.
Place the cod fish into a shallow, oiled baking dish.
Mix the tomatoes, olives, olive oil, garlic, and oregano in a bowl; pour over the cod.
Bake for about 12 to 14 minutes or until the fish is opaque and flakes easily when tested with a fork.
Serve and enjoy your dinner!

Nutrition Information (per serving):

Calories: 250, Protein: 31g, Carbs: 6g, Fiber: 2g, Fat: 10g, Cholesterol: 65mg, Sodium: 320mg, Potassium: 320mg.

Recipe 82: Zesty Baked trout

Prep. time: 8 min | Cook time: 20 min | Serves: 4

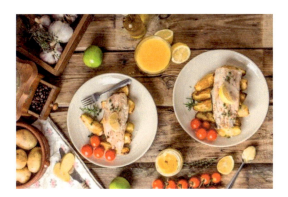

Directions:

Preheat your oven to 400°F.

Prepare a baking sheet by covering it with foil.

Combine the olive oil, lemon juice, garlic, parsley, salt, and pepper in a small bowl.

Place trout fillets on a prepared baking sheet and brush with the lemon garlic mixture.

Bake for 12-15 minutes or until the flesh of the trout becomes opaque and easily separates into flakes

Ingredients:

4 (6oz) trout fillets
1/4-cup olive oil
1/4 cup Lemon juice
4 minced cloves of garlic
2 tablespoons freshly chopped parsley
Salt and pepper to taste.

Nutritional Information (per serving):

Calories: 390, Protein: 32g, Carbs: 14g, Fiber: 3g, Fat: 23g, Cholesterol: 130mg, Sodium: 260mg, Potassium: 620mg.

Recipe 83: Macadamia Nut Crusted Mahi Mahi

Prep. time: 12 min | Cook time: 20 min | Serves: 3

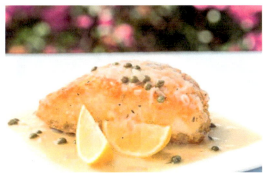

Directions:

Preheat your oven to 400°F. Line a baking sheet with foil.

In a shallow bowl, mix the chopped macadamia nuts and panko.

Dip the mahi in the egg and then in the nut coating to coat both sides. Then, move the pieces to a baking sheet and drizzle with olive oil, salt, and pepper.

Bake for 10 minutes, until the fish is opaque, and the nut crust is golden brown.

Serve and enjoy your dinner!

Ingredients:

4 (6 oz) mahi fillets
1 cup macadamia nuts, finely chopped
1/4 cup of panko breadcrumbs
2 large eggs, beaten
1 tablespoon olive oil
Salt and peppers to taste.

Nutritional Information (per serving):

Calories: 374, Protein: 24g, Carbs: 13g, Fiber: 4g, Fat: 22g, Cholesterol: 110mg, Sodium: 170mg, Potassium: 245mg.

Recipe 84: Steamed Halibut

Prep. time: 5 min | Cook time: 10 min | Serves: 3-4

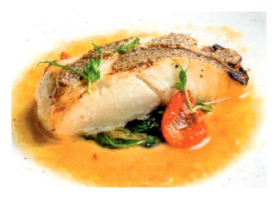

Directions:

Combine the vinegar, sesame oil, ginger, and garlic.
Place the halibut in a steamer basket and brush with the mixture. Steam for 8-10 minutes or until the fish is cooked through.
Serve and enjoy your dish!

Nutrition Information (per serving):

Calories: 220, Fat: 8g, Carbs: 1g, Fiber: 0g, Protein: 34g, Sodium: 85mg, Potassium: 700mg.

Ingredients:

4 (6 oz) Halibut fillets
2 tablespoons rice vinegar
1 tablespoon of sesame oil
1 tablespoon fresh ginger, grated
2 cloves garlic, minced
2 scallions
1/4 teaspoon of ground black pepper.

Recipe 85: Spicy Grilled Tuna Steaks

Prep. time: 10 min | Cook time: 15 min | Serves: 3

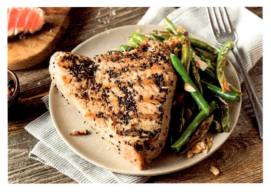

Directions:

Blend the olive oil, lime juice, and seasoning. Brush over the tuna steaks.
Grill for about 2-3 minutes per side to reach a medium-rare.
Serve and enjoy your dish!

Nutrition Information (per serving):

Calories: 232, Fat: 9g, Carbs: 3g, Fiber: 1.4g, Protein: 11g, Sodium: 90mg, Potassium: 460mg.

Ingredients:

4 (5-ounce) tuna
2 tablespoons olive oil
1 tablespoon lime juice
1 teaspoon paprika
1/2 teaspoon of cumin
1/4 teaspoon of cayenne
1/4 teaspoon of ground black pepper.

Recipe 86: Broiled mackerel with ginger and green onions

Prep. time: 8 min | Cook time: 20 min | Serves: 3

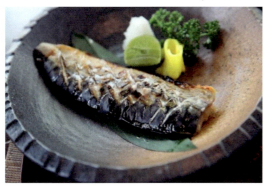

Directions:

Combine ginger, garlic, vinegar, and sesame oil.
Brush the mixtures onto mackerel fillets. Grill for about 4 to 5 minutes on each side.
Serve and enjoy your dish!=

Nutrition Information (per serving):

Calories: 280, Fat: 20g, Carbs: 2g, Fiber: 0g, Protein: 24g, Sodium: 85mg, Potassium: 500mg.

Ingredients:

4 (5 oz) mackerel fillets
2 tablespoons fresh ginger, grated
2 medium cloves garlic, minced
2 tablespoons rice vinegar
1 tablespoon of sesame oil
4 scallions
1/4 teaspoon of ground black pepper.

Recipe 87: Baked Cod

Prep. time: 10 min | Cook time: 20 min | Serves: 4

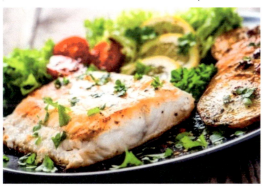

Directions:

Preheat the oven to 375°F (190°C). Place the cod in a baking dish and top with tomatoes and olives. Whisk the olive oil, lemon juice, garlic, and oregano in a small bowl. Drizzle over the fish.
Bake in the oven for 15-20 minutes until the fish is done.

Nutrition Information (per serving):

Calories: 250, Fat: 12g, Carbs: 4g, Fiber: 1g, Protein: 30g, Sodium: 200mg, Potassium: 800mg.

Ingredients:

4 (6 oz) cod fillets
1 cup cherry tomatoes, halved
1/4 cup Kalamata olives pitted
2 tablespoons of olive oil
2 tablespoons of lemon juice
2 cloves minced garlic
1 teaspoon dried oregano
1/4 teaspoon of black pepper.

Recipe 88: Pesto-crusted Sea Bass

Prep. time: 8 min | Cook time: 15 min | Serves: 4

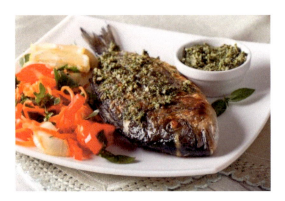

Ingredients:

4 (6 oz) fillets of sea bass
1/4 cup of homemade pesto: basil, olive oil,
garlic, pine nuts
2 tablespoons lemon juice
1/4 cup ground almonds
1/4 teaspoon of ground black pepper.

Directions:

Preheat the oven to 400°F (200°C).
 Mix the pesto with the lemon juice. Spread pesto mixture over fish fillets.
Top with almond flour and pepper.
Bake for 12-15 minutes or until fish is cooked through
Serve and enjoy your dish!

Nutrition Information (per serving):

Calories: 300, Fat: 18g, Carbs: 3g, Fiber: 1g, Protein: 32g,
Sodium: 120mg, Potassium: 550mg.

Recipe 89: Poached Flounder with Ginger

Prep. time: 10 min | Cook time: 10 min | Serves: 4-5

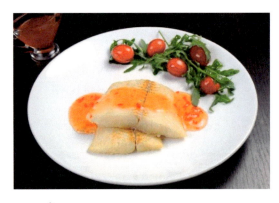

Ingredients:

4 (6 oz) fillets flounder
2 cups water
1/4 cup vinegar
1 tablespoon fresh ginger, grated
2 cloves garlic, minced
2 scallions.

Directions:

Bring the water, vinegar, ginger, and garlic to a boil in a large skillet.
Heat to a simmer over medium heat.
Add the flounder fillets and poach until fully cooked for 5-7 minutes.
Garnish with chopped scallions.
Serve and enjoy your dish!

Nutrition Information (per serving):

Calories: 300, Fat: 18g, Carbohydrates: 3g
Fiber: 1g, Protein: 32g, Sodium: 120mg
Potassium: 550mg.

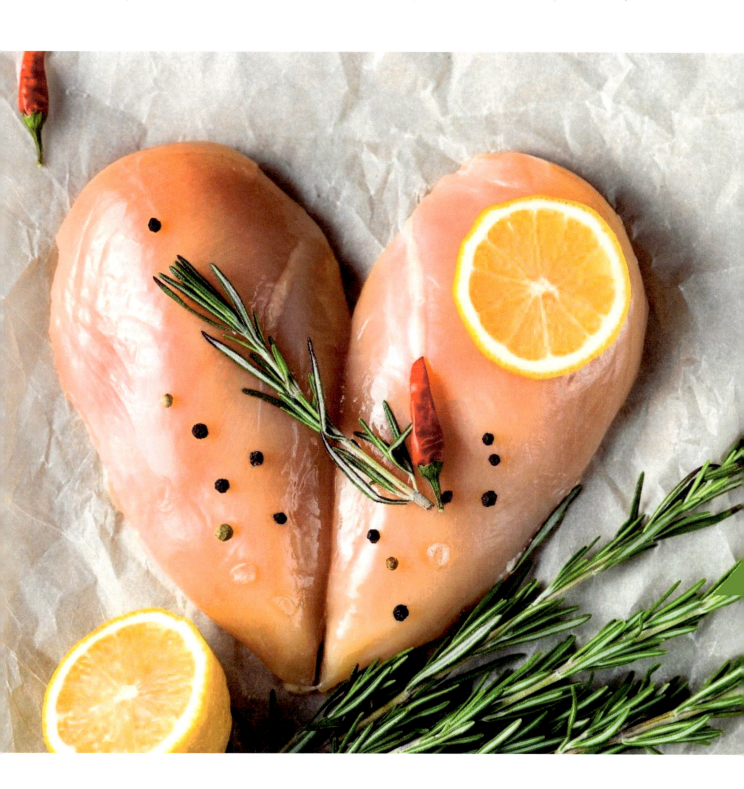

Recipe 90: Herb-crusted chicken breast

Prep. time: 10 min | Cook time: 30 min | Serves: 4

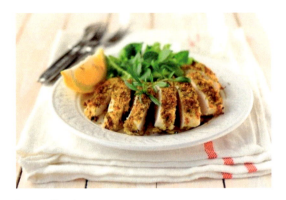

Directions:

Preheat your oven to a temperature of 400°F.
Lightly coat the baking dish with cooking spray.
Add the olive oil, thyme, rosemary, garlic powder, and pepper to a small bowl.
Rub the herb mixture over the chicken breast.
Add the chicken to a baking dish and roast for 25 to 30 minutes or until done.
Serve and enjoy your dinner!

Ingredients:

4 (6 oz) Chicken boneless, skinless
2 tablespoons olive oil
1 teaspoon thyme, dried
1 teaspoon of dried rosemary
1 teaspoon of garlic powder. Salt and pepper to taste.

Nutritional Information (per serving):

Calories: 220, Protein: 38g, Carbs: 1g, Fiber: 0g, Fat: 7g, Cholesterol: 105mg, Sodium: 150mg, Potassium: 470mg.

Recipe 91: Citrus Grilled Chicken

Prep. time: 10 min | Cook time: 150 min | Serves: 3-4

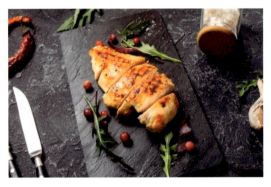

Directions:

Whisk together all the marinade ingredients except the chicken. Marinate the chicken for 2 hours.
Grill for 6-8 minutes per side until cooked through.

Nutrition information (per serving):

Calories: 240, Fat: 10g, Carbs: 3g, Fiber: 0g, Protein: 34g, Sodium: 70mg, Potassium: 400mg.

Ingredients:

4 (6 oz) boneless, skinless chicken breasts
2 tablespoons of olive oil
2 tablespoons of orange juice
1 tablespoon of lemon juice
1 tablespoon of lime juice
1 teaspoon of honey
1 Clove garlic minced
1/4 teaspoon of black pepper.

Recipe 92: Turkey Veggie Lettuce Wraps

Prep. time: 15 min | Cook time: 10 min | Serves: 4

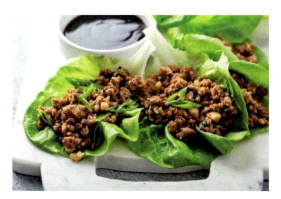

Ingredients:

1 Pound of lean ground turkey
1 red bell pepper
1 Cup Mushrooms, sliced
2 scallions, chopped
2 garlic cloves minced
2 tablespoons low-sodium soy sauce
8 large lettuce leaves.

Directions:

Brown and crumble the ground turkey in a skillet over medium-high heat.
Add the bell pepper, mushrooms, green onions, and garlic Cook for 3 to 4 minutes.
Add the soy sauce and cook for 1 more minute
Fill the leaves with the turkey-veggie mixture
Serve and enjoy your dinner!

Nutritional information (per serving):

Calories: 180, Protein: 26g, Carbs: 6g, Fiber: 2g, Fat: 5g, Cholesterol: 80mg, Sodium: 250mg, Potassium: 610mg.

Recipe 93: Baked Pesto Turkey Meatballs

Prep. time: 10 min | Cook time: 25 min | Serves: 4-5

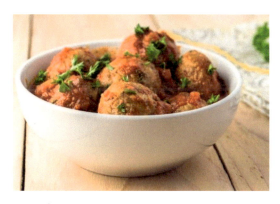

Ingredients:

1 lb ground turkey
1/4 cup homemade pesto (basil, olive oil, garlic, pine nuts)
1/4-cup almond flour
1 egg 1/4 teaspoon ground black pepper.

Directions:

Preheat the oven to 375°F (190°C). Put all the ingredients into the bowl.
Shape into 16 meatballs.
Bake for 20 to 25 minutes or until done
Serve and enjoy your dish!

Nutrition information (per 4 meatballs): Calories:

280, Fat: 20g, Carbs: 3g, Fiber: 1g, Protein: 24g, Sodium: 80mg, Potassium: 300mg.

Recipe 94: Grilled Spicy (moderate) Chicken Skewers

Prep. time: 10 min | Cook time: 15 min | Serves: 4

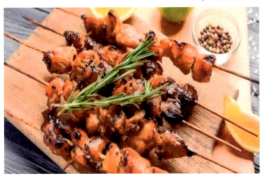

Ingredients:

1 lb boneless, skinless chicken breasts cut into cubes
2 tablespoons olive oil
1 tablespoon lime juice
1 tsp Paprika
1 tsp cumin
1/2 tsp Cayenne pepper
1/4 tsp black pepper.

Directions:

Mix olive oil, lime juice, and spices.
Marinate chicken cubes for 30 minutes.
Thread onto skewers and grill for 10-12 minutes, turning occasionally.
Serve and enjoy!

Nutrition information (per serving, 4 servings total):

Calories: 220, Fat: 11g, Carbs: 1g, Fiber: 0g, Protein: 28g, Sodium: 60mg, Potassium: 350mg.

Recipe 95: Chicken Masala

Prep. time: 10 min | Cook time: 30 min | Serves: 2-4

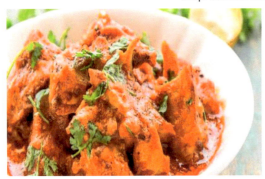

Ingredients:

1 tablespoon of avocado oil
1 tablespoon of diced ginger
1 tablespoon of minced jalapeño peppers
1 Pound of boneless chicken thighs, skinless
½ Cup of chopped tomatoes
1 tsp of turmeric
½ tsp of spices of your choice (cumin, chili...)
½ tsp of cayenne
¼ Cup of chopped cilantro

Directions:

Heat your saucepan. Spray your saucepan with vegetarian cooking oil spray.
Add the jalapeno pepper and the ginger.
Add in the chicken and the tomatoes, and stir
Add the spices, 1 tablespoon of sesame oil, and ½ water.
Cover your ingredients and cook them for about 29 minutes.
Pour in a deep salad bowl everything.
Garnish with coriander or mint leaves.
Serve, and enjoy your dish!

Nutrition information (per 4 meatballs):

Calories: 301, Fat: 14g, Carbs: 12g, Fiber: 2.1g, Protein: 16g, Sodium: 65mg, Potassium: 250mg.

Recipe 96: Stuffed Chicken

Prep. time: 15 min | Cook time: 25 min | Serves: 3

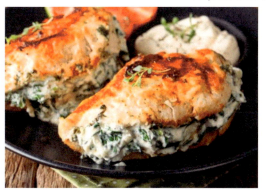

Ingredients:

2 whole chicken breasts
1 large onion
1 large tomato
1 large capsicum
1 large eggplant
1 teaspoon tahini paste
Chili powder to taste
1 Tablespoon of olive oil.

Directions:

Place the chicken breasts flat and hit it using a meat tenderizer. Set it aside.

Place the capsicum and eggplants on open flames and allow the skin to char. It takes about 10-15 minutes to char, and make sure you turn the vegetables every 5 minutes. Once they char, run them under water and allow the skin to wash off. Place the vegetables in a bowl, add the oil, tahini paste, chili powder, and mix well. Add chopped onion and tomatoes to the mix and mix well.

Place half the mix on one breast and the other half on the other breast, and fold both sides of each breast inwards to make an envelope. Place the breasts in a pre-heated 390° F oven for 20-25 minutes.

Nutrition information (per serving, 4 servings total):

Calories: 289, Fat: 10.4g, Carbs: 4g, Fiber: 1.2, Protein: 11g, Sodium: 40mg, Potassium: 280mg.

Recipe 97: Chicken breasts with mango and pineapple

Prep. time: 10 min | Cook time: 40 min | Serves: 4

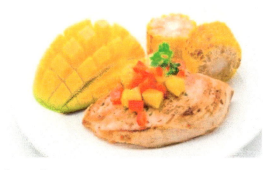

Ingredients:

2 chicken breasts (skinned and boned)
2 Tablespoons of pineapple juice
1 and ½ teaspoons of minced ginger
2 Minced garlic pods
1 Pinch of salt to taste
1 Pinch of fresh black pepper
2 Cups of diced mango
½ Cup of milk
Freshly chopped cilantro.
1 tablespoon of lemon juice.

Directions:

Place the chicken breasts in a bowl, and add the minced ginger, garlic pods, salt, and pepper. Please give it a good mix and set it aside for 30 minutes. Meanwhile, dice the mango into cubes and place it in the milk. Preheat oven to 480 degrees Fahrenheit, place the chicken breasts, and bake for 40 minutes. Allow the chicken to cool before mixing with the mango and coconut mix. Serve with a sprinkling of cilantro on top.

Nutrition information (per 4 meatballs):

Calories: 333, Fat: 12g, Carbs: 11g, Fiber: 2.4g, Protein: 13g, Sodium: 76mg, Potassium: 280mg.

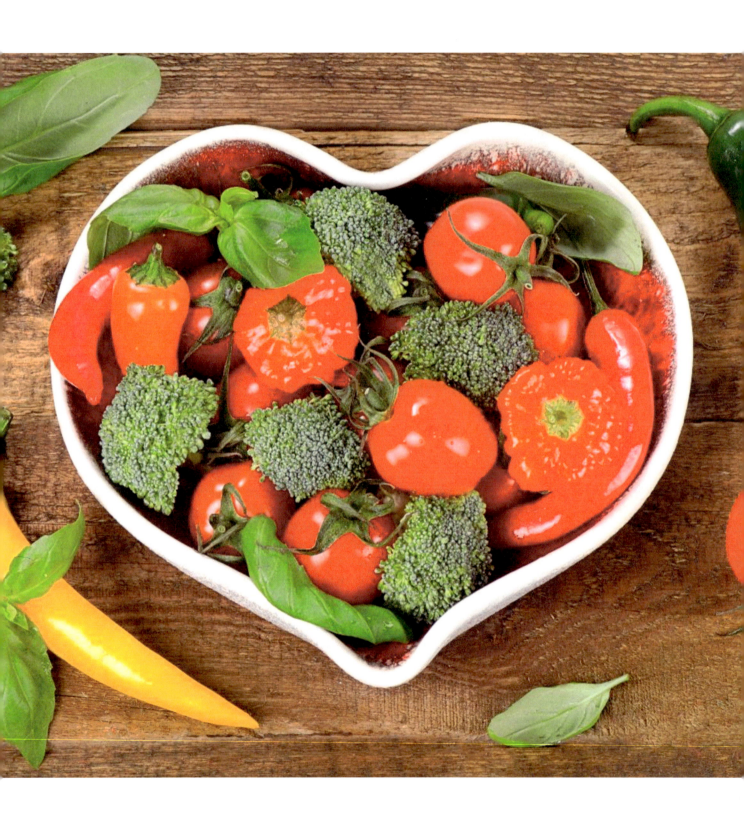

Recipe 98: Veggie Tacos

Prep. time: 12 min | Cook time: 15 min | Serves:

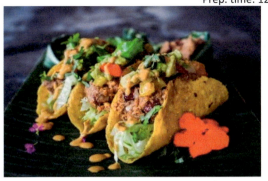

Ingredients:

1 cup of cooked black beans, very well rinsed and drained, 1 cup of cooked lentils
1 cup of chopped bell peppers
1 cup of diced zucchini, 1/2 cup of diced red onion, 2 Finely minced Garlic Cloves
1 teaspoon of ground cumin
1 teaspoon of chili powder
1/4 teaspoon of smoked paprika
2 tablespoons of chopped fresh cilantro
8 small corn tortillas, 1 Medium sliced avocado
Lime wedges for garnish.

Directions:

Brown and crumble the ground turkey in a skillet over medium-high heat.
Add the bell pepper, mushrooms, green onions, and garlic Cook for 3 to 4 minutes.
Add the soy sauce and cook for 1 more minute
Fill the leaves with the turkey-veggie mixture
Serve and enjoy your dinner!

Nutrition information (per serving):

Calories: 280, Protein: 12g, Carbs: 39g, Fiber: 8g, Fat: 10g, Cholesterol: 0mg, Sodium: 180mg, Potassium: 520mg.

Recipe 99: Le'ntil Walnut Veggie Burgers

Prep. time: 14 min | Cook time: 15 min | Serves: 6

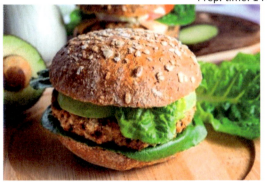

Ingredients:

1 cup of cooked lentils
1 cup of chopped walnuts
1 cup of oat flour
1 grated carrot
½ diced onion
2 minced garlic cloves
1 flax egg (1 tablespoon of ground flax + 3 tablespoons of water)
1 teaspoon of dried thyme
Salt and pepper to taste
6 whole wheat buns.

Directions:

In a bowl, mash the lentils lightly.
Mix walnuts, oat flour, carrot, onion, garlic, flax egg, thyme, salt and pepper.
Form your mixture into 6 patties.
Cook your patties in a skillet over medium heat for 5 minutes per side until browned.
Serve on whole wheat buns with desired toppings.
Enjoy your veggie burgers!

Nutrition information (per 4 meatballs):

Calories: 244, Protein: 8.3g, Carbs: 22g, Fiber: 2.1g, Fat: 1.1g, Cholesterol: 0mg, Sodium: 39mg, Potassium: 390mg.

Recipe 100: Cauliflower Gnocchi

Prep. time: 10min | Cook time: 15 min | Serves: 4

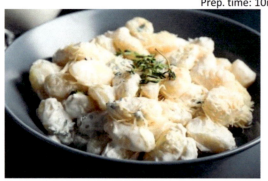

Ingredients:

1 large head cauliflower, separated
into florets (about 6 cups)
1 cup almond meal, 1/2 cup grated parmesan
cheese, 1 large egg
1 teaspoon of garlic powder
1/2 teaspoon salt, 1/4 teaspoon black pepper,
2 tablespoons olive oil
1 cup marinara sauce (low sodium)
Fresh basil leaves to garnish.

Directions:

Brown and crumble the ground turkey in a skillet over
medium-high heat.
Add the bell pepper, mushrooms, green onions, and garlic.
Cook for 3 to 4 minutes.
Add the soy sauce and cook for 1 more minute.
Fill the leaves with the turkey-veggie mixture.
Serve and enjoy your dinner!

Nutritional information (per serving):

Calories: 283, Protein: 10.4g, Carbs: 13g, Fiber: 7g, Fat: 18g,
Cholesterol: 43mg, Sodium: 150mg, Potassium: 420mg.

Recipe 101: Chickpea and Cauliflower Curry

Prep. time: 15 min | Cook time: 10 min | Serves: 6

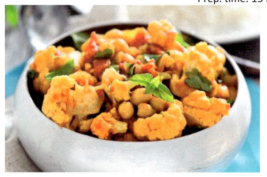

Ingredients:

1 large head of cauliflower
broken into florets, 2 cans (15 oz each) of no-
salt-added chickpeas, rinsed and drained
1 onion, chopped, 3 cloves garlic, minced
1 tablespoon fresh ginger, grated
2 tablespoons olive oil, 2 tablespoons curry
powder, 1 teaspoon ground cumin
1/2 teaspoon of turmeric, 1/4 teaspoon of
cayenne pepper, 1 (14-ounce) can no-salt-
added diced tomatoes, 1 (14-ounce) can light
coconut milk, 2 cups fresh spinach
1/4 cup Fresh Cilantro
1/4 tsp black pepper
The juice of 1 lime.

Directions:

Heat olive oil in a large pot over medium heat. Add onion,
garlic, and ginger, cooking for about 5 minutes until the onion
softens. Stir in curry powder, cumin, turmeric, and cayenne (if
using), and cook for another minute.
Add cauliflower florets and chickpeas, mixing well to coat with
spices. Stir in diced tomatoes and coconut milk, bring to a
simmer, then reduce to low heat. Cover and cook for 15-20
minutes, stirring occasionally, until the cauliflower is tender.
Add spinach and cook until wilted, about 2-3 minutes. Turn off
the heat and stir in fresh cilantro, black pepper, and lime juice.
Let stand for 5 minutes before serving. Serve over brown rice
or with whole-grain naan bread, if desired.

Nutrition information (per serving, 6 servings total):

Calories: 280, Fat: 12g, Carbs: 36g, Fiber: 11g, Protein: 11g,
Sodium: 60mg, Potassium: 700mg.

Recipe 102: Quinoa Bowl

Prep. time: 15 min | Cook time:25 min | Serves: 4

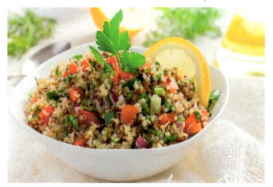

Ingredients:

1 cup quinoa, rinsed, 2 cups water
1 medium sweet potato, diced
1 Red Bell Pepper, Sliced
1 zucchini, sliced, 1 red onion, cut into
wedges, 2 tablespoons olive oil
1 tsp dried thyme, 1 teaspoon dried
rosemary, 1/4 tsp black pepper, 1 can (15 oz)
no-salt-added chickpeas, rinsed and drained,
2 cups fresh spinach
1/4 cup tahini, 2 tablespoons lemon juice
1 clove garlic, minced. Water.

Directions:

Preheat the oven to 400°F (200°C). Cook the quinoa: Bring to a boil, reduce heat, cover, and simmer for 15-20 minutes until the water is absorbed. Fluff with a fork. Place sweet potato, bell pepper, zucchini, and red onion on a baking sheet. Drizzle with 1 tbsp olive oil, sprinkle with thyme, rosemary, and black pepper, and stir. Roast for 20-25 minutes, stirring halfway. Toss chickpeas with 1 tbsp olive oil and add for 10 minutes.

Mix tahini, lemon juice, and minced garlic, thinning with water for dressing. Assemble bowls with quinoa, roasted veggies, chickpeas, fresh spinach, and tahini dressing. Serve and enjoy!

Nutritional information (per serving):

Calories: 285, Protein: 12g, Carbs: 39g, Fiber: 8g, Fat: 10g, Cholesterol: 0mg, Sodium: 180mg, Potassium: 520mg.

Recipe 103: Stuffed Eggplant

Prep. time: 14 min | Cook time: 10 min | Serves: 3-4

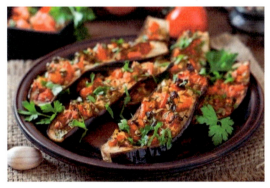

Ingredients:

2 medium-sized eggplants
1 cup green lentils, rinsed
2 cups of water 1 onion, finely minced
2 cloves garlic, minced 1 red bell pepper,
diced 1 zucchini, diced
1 (14 oz) can of diced tomatoes with no salt
2 tablespoons olive oil
1 teaspoon of dried oregano
1 teaspoon of dried basil
1/4 cup chopped fresh parsley
1/4 cup crumbled light feta cheese
1/4 teaspoon ground black pepper.

Directions:

Preheat your oven to 375°F (190°C). Halve the eggplants lengthwise. Scoop the pulp from each half, leaving a 1/2-inch-thick border. Coarsely dice the scooped pulp; set aside. For lentils: Bring lentils and water to boil in a medium saucepan. Reduce heat and simmer, uncovered, until tender, 20-25 minutes. Drain away any leftover cooking water—heat olive oil in a large skillet over medium heat. Add onion and garlic and sauté for 3–4 minutes until lentils are cooked. Add the eggplant pulp, bell pepper, and zucchini. Cook for 5–7 minutes until the vegetables are tender. Add cooked lentils, diced tomatoes, oregano, and basil. Let it simmer for 5 minutes. Remove from heat and mix in the parsley and black pepper. Fill eggplant halves with lentil filling; place the eggplants in a baking dish. Bake for 30-35 minutes, covered in foil. Remove the foil, sprinkle the feta cheese, and bake an extra 10 minutes uncovered.

Nutritional information (based on one stuffed eggplant half):

Calories 283, Fat 9g, Carbohydrates 40g, Fiber 16g, Protein 14g, Sodium 110mg, Potassium 900mg.

Recipe 104: Vegetable and Tofu Stir-Fry

Prep. time: 8 min | Cook time: 15 min | Serves: 4

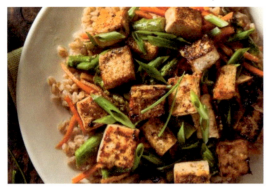

Ingredients:

1 block (14 oz) extra-firm tofu, pressed and cubed, 2 tablespoons low-sodium soy sauce
1 tablespoon cornstarch, 2 tablespoons sesame oil, 2 cloves garlic, minced
1 tablespoon ginger, fresh, grated
1 crown of broccoli, floret
1 red bell pepper, julienned
1carrot, julienned, 1 cup snap peas, 1/4 cup vegetable stock, 1 tbsp rice vinegar, 1 teaspoon honey, 1/4 cup peanuts, chopped
2 green onions, chopped.

Directions:

 Toss together tofu, one tablespoon of soy sauce, and cornstarch. Heat one tablespoon of sesame oil in a large wok or skillet and brown the tofu over medium heat until crispy. Remove and set aside. Heat the remaining oil in the same pan, add the garlic and ginger, and cook for 30 seconds. Add vegetables and stir-fry for 5-7. Add the remaining soy sauce, broth, vinegar, and honey. Pour in and let simmer for 2 minutes. Return tofu to the pan and heat through. Sprinkle with peanuts and green onions.

Nutritional Information (per serving):

Calories: 270, Protein: 14g, Carbs: 22g, Fiber: 3g, Fat: 15g, Cholesterol: 0mg, Sodium: 260mg, Potassium: 570mg.

Recipe 105: Lentil and Vegetable Loaf

Prep. time: 10 min | Cook time: 45 min | Serves: 3-4

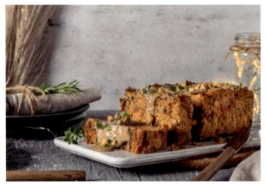

Ingredients:

1 cup dried green lentils
2 1/2 cups water, 1 tablespoon of olive oil
1 Onion, finely chopped
2 carrots, grated, 2 celery sticks, finely chopped, 2 cloves garlic, minced, 1 cup Mushrooms, minced, 1 Cup rolled oats
1/4 cup ground flax, 1/4 cup tomato paste
1 teaspoon dried thyme
1 teaspoon dried rosemary
1/4 teaspoon of ground black pepper.

Directions:

Cook the lentils in water until cooked but not overdone, 20-25 minutes. Drain and mash a bit.
Preheat the oven to 375°F (190°C). Sauté onion, carrots, celery, garlic, and mushrooms in olive oil for about 5-7 minutes.
Mix the lentils, sautéed vegetables, rolled oats, flaxseed, tomato paste, herbs, and pepper well in a large bowl. Press into a loaf pan lined with parchment paper. Bake for 40-45 minutes until the mixture and a light brown crust have been set. Let it cool for 10 minutes before slicing.
Serve and enjoy your dish!

Nutrition information (per serving):

Calories: 250, Protein: 13g, Carbs: 40g, Fiber: 12g, Fat: 6g, Cholesterol: 0mg, Sodium: 140mg, Potassium: 620mg.

Recipe 106: Vegetarian Moussaka

Prep. time: 12 min | Cook time: 50 min | Serves: 3-4

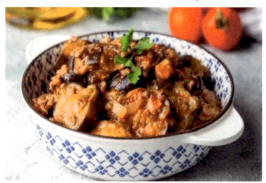

Ingredients:

2 large eggplants, sliced, 1 tablespoon olive oil, 1 onion, diced 2 cloves garlic, minced 1 can (14 oz) no-salt-added diced tomatoes 1 cup cooked lentils 1 teaspoon dried oregano ½ teaspoon floor cinnamon 1/four teaspoon black pepper For the topping: 2 cups almond milk, 1/4 cup whole wheat flour, 1/four cup grated Parmesan cheese 2 eggs, beaten, 1/4 teaspoon nutmeg.

Directions:

Preheat oven to 375°F (190°C).
Grill or roast eggplant slices until everything becomes tender.
In a pan, sauté onion and garlic in olive oil.
Add tomatoes, lentils, oregano, cinnamon, and pepper. Simmer for 10 mins.
Layer eggplant and lentil in a baking dish.
Topping, whisk the almond milk and almond flour in a saucepan over medium heat until thickening.
Remove from heat, stir in Parmesan, eggs, and nutmeg.
Pour topping over layered eggplant and lentils.
Bake for 35-40 minutes till golden brown.
Serve and enjoy your dish!

Nutritional Information (in keeping with serving):

Calories: 298, Protein: 17g, Carbs: 30g, Fiber: 10g, Fat: 10.3g, Cholesterol: 78mg, Sodium: 130mg, Potassium: 570mg.

Recipe 107: Vegetable and Tofu Kebabs with Peanut Sauce

Prep. time: 10 min | Cook time: 12 min | Serves: 3

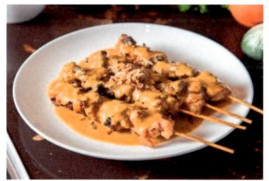

Ingredients:

1 block (14 oz) extra-firm tofu, cubed
1 red bell pepper, cut into chunks
1 zucchini, sliced thick, 1 red onion, cut into wedges, 8 cherry tomatoes 2 tablespoons olive oil, 1teaspoon dried thyme, 1/4 teaspoon ground black pepper
For the sauce:
1/4 cup natural peanut butter
1 tablespoon of lime juice 1 tablespoon honey 1clove garlic, minced
1/4 teaspoon red pepper flakes.

Directions:

Preheat your grill or grill pan to medium-high heat. Toss together tofu, peppers, mushrooms, zucchini, olive oil, thyme, and pepper in a medium bowl.
Thread on skewers. Grill for 10 to 12 minutes or until vegetables are tender, turning occasionally.
Whisk all ingredients together for the sauce and thin with water if needed. Serve kebabs with peanut sauce for dipping.

Nutritional information (per serving):

Calories: 270, Protein: 11g, Carbs: 13g, Fiber: 2g, Fat: 9g, Cholesterol: 15mg, Sodium: 98mg, Potassium: 340mg.

Recipe 108: Cauliflower Wellington

Prep. time: 30min | Cook time: 40min | Serves: 6

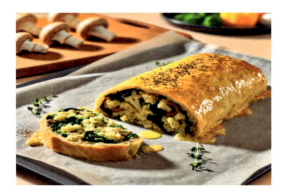

Ingredients :

1 head of cauliflower broken into florets
2 tablespoons of olive oil
1 chopped onion
3 minced cloves of garlic
1 cup of mushrooms slices
1 cup of chopped spinach
1/2 cup of almond flour
1/2 cup of grated parmesan cheese
2 large eggs
1 teaspoon of dry thyme
1/2 teaspoon salt
1/4 teaspoon black pepper
4 oz of softening cream cheese
1 package (7-8 ounces) puff pastry or
fathead dough.

Directions:

Preheat the oven to 400°F (200°C). Steam or boil cauliflower florets until tender, about 8-10 minutes. Drain and let cool. Sauté onion and garlic in olive oil over medium heat for 2 minutes, then add mushrooms and spinach, cooking for 5 minutes until soft. Remove from heat and cool. Pulse cauliflower in a food processor to breadcrumb consistency. Combine cauliflower, almond flour, Parmesan, eggs, thyme, salt, and pepper in a large bowl. Add the sautéed vegetables and cream cheese, mixing well. Roll out puff pastry on a parchment-lined baking sheet, placing the cauliflower mixture in the center as a log. Fold dough over the mixture, crimping edges. Brush with beaten egg or olive oil. Bake for 30-35 minutes until golden brown. Serve and enjoy your dinner!

Nutritional Information (per serving):

Calories: 320, Protein: 14g, Carbs: 12g, Fiber: 4g, Fat: 24g, Cholesterol: 120mg, Sodium: 450mg, Potassium: 550mg

CHAPTER 6: SIDES AND ACCOMPANIMENTS

6.1. VIBRANT VEGETABLE DISHES

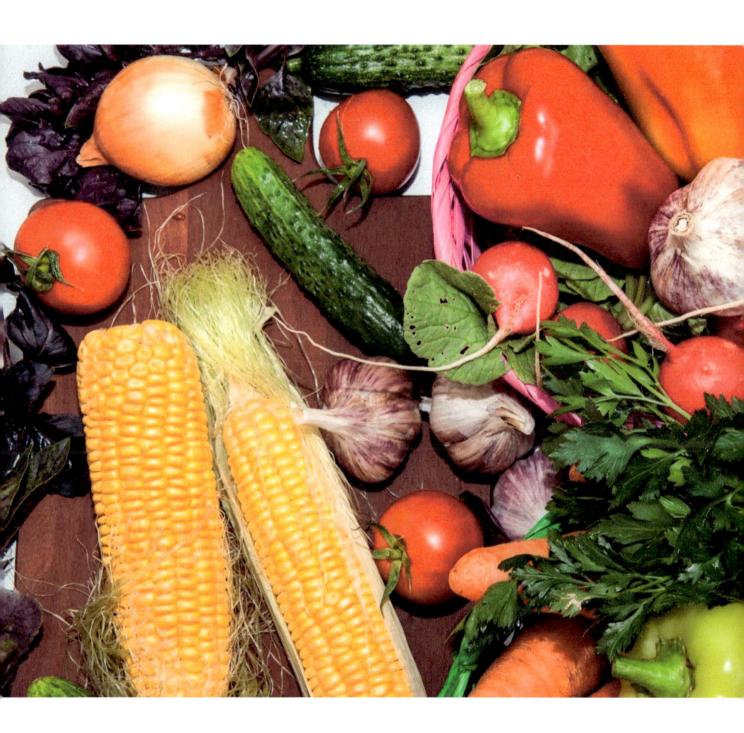

Recipe 109: Smashed Zucchini with Pesto & Burrata

Prep. time: 13 min | Cook time: 11 min | Serves: 3-4

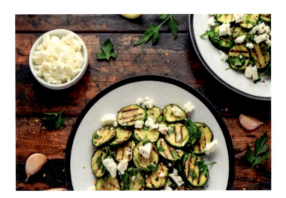

Ingredients:

4 medium zucchini - halved lengthwise
2 tablespoons olive oil, 1 clove garlic,
minced, 1/4 teaspoon black pepper
1/2 cup fresh basil leaves
2 tablespoons pine nuts, toasted
2 tablespoons grated Parmesan cheese
1 tablespoon lemon juice, 2 tablespoons
olive oil for pesto, 8 ounces burrata cheese,
Lemon wedges to serve.

Directions:

Preheat the oven to 400°F (200°C). Place the zucchini halves cut side up on a baking sheet. Drizzle with 2 tbsp olive oil, sprinkle with minced garlic, and black pepper. Roast for 10-12 minutes until tender.

Meanwhile, make pesto by blending basil leaves, pine nuts, Parmesan cheese, lemon juice, and 2 tbsp olive oil to a coarse paste.

Remove zucchini from the oven, smash with a fork, top with burrata cheese, and drizzle with pesto. Serve with lemon wedges.

Nutritional information (per serving):

Calories: 270, Protein: 11g, Carbs: 11g, Fiber: 2.3g, Fat: 17g, Cholesterol: 30mg, Sodium: 204mg, Potassium: 450mg.

Recipe 110: Grilled Corn and Black Bean Salsa

Prep. time: 20min | Cook time: 15 min | Serves: 6

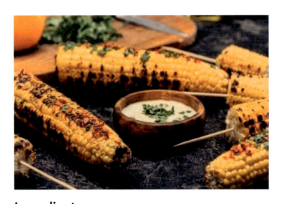

Ingredients:

4 ears of corn, husks removed
1 (15 oz) can black beans, rinsed and
drained, 1 red bell pepper, diced
1/2 red onion, diced
1 jalapeno, seeded and minced
1/4 cup fresh cilantro, chopped
2 tablespoons lime juice
1 tablespoon olive oil
1/2 teaspoon salt
1/4 teaspoon black pepper.

Directions:

Preheat the grill to medium-high heat.

Grill the corn, turning occasionally, until charred in spots, about 10-12 minutes. Let the grilled corn cool slightly, then remove the kernels from the cobs. Combine the corn kernels, black beans, red bell pepper, red onion, jalapeno, and cilantro in a large bowl.

Whisk together the lime juice, olive oil, salt, and black pepper in a small bowl.

Pour the dressing over the corn and bean mixture and toss gently to combine.

Serve the salsa at room temperature or chilled, with tortilla chips or as a topping for tacos or salads.

Nutritional Information (per serving):

Calories: 140, Protein: 6g, Carbs: 25g, Fiber: 6g, Fat: 3g, Cholesterol: 0mg, Sodium: 280mg, Potassium: 430mg.

Recipe 111: Balsamic Glazed Roasted Root Vegetables

Prep. time: 10 min | Cook time: 40 min | Serves: 3-4

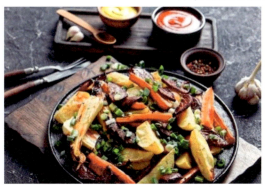

Ingredients:

4 medium zucchini - halved lengthwise
2 tablespoons olive oil, 1 clove garlic,
minced, 1/4 teaspoon black pepper
1/2 cup fresh basil leaves
2 tablespoons pine nuts, toasted
2 tablespoons grated Parmesan cheese
1 tablespoon lemon juice
2 tablespoons olive oil for pesto
8 ounces burrata cheese
Lemon wedges to serve.

Directions:

Preheat your oven to 200°C (400).
Toss sweet potato, parsnips, and beets in a large bowl.
Combine the olive oil, balsamic vinegar, and rosemary in a small bowl.
Pour the sauce on the vegetables and toss lightly to mix well.
Spread the vegetables in a single layer on a cookie sheet.
Bake, stirring every 10 minutes or so, until the vegetables are tender and golden brown, 35 to 40 minutes.
Serve and enjoy your dish!

Nutritional information (per serving, serves 4):

Calories: 120, Protein: 2g, Carbs: 22g, Fiber: 4g, Fat: 3.5g,
Sodium: 65mg, Potassium: 450mg.

Recipe 112: Herb Roasted Portabella Mushrooms

Prep. time: 5 min | Cook time: 25 min | Serves: 1-2

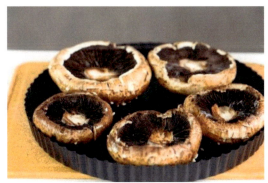

Ingredients:

4 large portobello mushrooms, stems removed
2 tablespoons olive oil
2 garlic cloves, minced
1 tablespoon of chopped fresh thyme leaves
1 tablespoon of fresh rosemary, chopped
1/4 teaspoon of black pepper, ground.

Directions:

Preheat the oven to 375°F (190. Clean mushrooms and remove the stems.
Mix the minced garlic, thyme, rosemary, and black pepper into the olive oil.
Brush both sides of the mushrooms with the herb mixture. Arrange the mushrooms with gill sides up on a baking sheet. Roast for 20-25 minutes until the mushrooms are tender. Slice and serve as a savory, vegetarian side.

Nutritional information (per serving, serves 4):

Calories: 90, Protein: 3g, Carbs: 5g, Fiber: 2g, Fat: 7g
Sodium: 30mg, Potassium: 250mg.

Recipe 113: Curried Eggplants

Prep. time: 8 min | Cook time: 40 min | Serves: 3-4

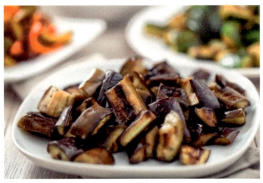

Ingredients:

1 large eggplant
2 tbsp of vegetable oil
1 Teaspoon of cumin seeds
1 medium onion, minced
1/2 tsp of grated fresh ginger
1/2 tsp of crushed garlic
1 teaspoon of curry powder
1 tomato, diced
1/2 cup of plain yogurt
1 hot jalapeño pepper, finely chopped
1 teaspoon of salt
1/4 bunch of chopped fresh cilantro.

Directions:

Preheat the oven to 450 ° F (230 ° C).
Place the eggplant on a baking sheet and cook until tender, 20 to 30 minutes. Remove it from the oven and let it cool so it can be peeled and cut into pieces.
Heat the oil in a skillet. Add the cumin and onion and sauté until the onion is tender. Add the ginger, garlic, curry, and tomato and cook for 1 minute. Then, add the yogurt. Mix with the eggplant and chili and season with salt. Cover and cook for 10 minutes over medium-high heat.
Remove the lid, reduce the heat to low, and then simmer for 5 minutes.
Garnish with the cilantro, then serve and enjoy your dish!

Nutritional Information (per serving, serves 4):

Calories: 140, Protein: 4g, Carbs: 15g, Fiber: 2g, Fat: 2.1g, Sodium: 56mg, Potassium: 357mg.

Recipe114: Kale Dip

Prep. time: 10 min | Cook time: 10 min | Serves: 3

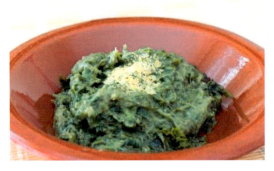

Ingredients:

½ Head of purple-green or Dino chopped kale
½ Tablespoon of extra-virgin olive oil
½ Cup of raw organic sesame seeds
¼ Cup of extra-virgin olive oil
4 Green onions, only the green part
1 ½ Tablespoons of apple cider vinegar
1 Pinch of grey sea salt.

Directions:

Add the chopped kale and 1 tablespoon of olive oil to a large cast iron pan and heat on low heat for about 7 minutes. Transfer to a food processor with an 'S' blade. Add the remaining ingredients and blend until smooth. Spoon into the Mason jar and store in the refrigerator for about 4 to 5 days!
Serve and enjoy your dish!

Nutritional information (per serving, serves 4):

Calories: 97, Protein: 2.4g, Carbs: 9g, Fiber: 3g, Fat: 3g, Sodium: 60mg, Potassium: 214mg.

Recipe 115: Avocado Mash

Prep. time: 5 min | Cook time: 10 min | Serves: 2

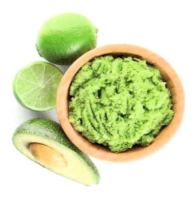

Ingredients:

1 Cup of unsalted macadamia nuts
1 Large avocado
1 Garlic clove
1 Tablespoon of tahini paste
½ Teaspoon of sea salt
2 Tablespoons of fresh lime juice
2 Tablespoons of extra virgin olive oil
Chopped fresh cilantro.

Directions:

Place the macadamia nuts in a container, then fill it with water. Let soak at room temperature for about 2 hours or overnight.

Strain and rinse the macadamia nuts after soaking; then discard the liquid.

Peel the avocado and remove the seed; then peel the garlic and slice it.

Add chopped fresh cilantro.

Put your ingredients in a food processor, then process until your ingredients become smooth.

Transfer to a bowl; then drizzle the olive oil on top and garnish with cilantro leaves.

Serve with freshly chopped vegetables like carrots, celery sticks, and peppers.

Nutritional information (per serving, serves 4):

Calories: 152, Protein: 3g, Carbs: 12g, Fiber: 1.3g, Fat: 2.3g, Sodium: 46mg, Potassium: 230mg.

Recipe 116: Garlic Roasted Green Beans

Prep. time: 10 min | Cook time: 10 min | Serves: 4

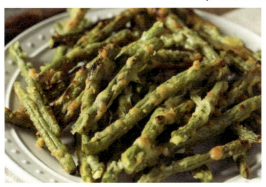

Ingredients:

1-pound fresh green beans, trimmed
2 tablespoons olive oil
4 cloves garlic, minced
1/2 teaspoon dried thyme
1/4 teaspoon salt
1/4 teaspoon black pepper
2 tablespoons grated Parmesan cheese (optional).

Directions:

Preheat the oven to 400°F (200°C).

In a large bowl, toss the green beans with olive oil, minced garlic, dried thyme, salt, and black pepper until well coated.

Spread the green beans onto a large baking sheet in a single layer.

Roast for 18-20 minutes, stirring occasionally, until the green beans are tender and lightly browned.

Remove from the oven and sprinkle with grated Parmesan cheese (if using).

Serve hot and enjoy your side.

Nutritional Information (per serving):

Calories: 100, Protein: 2g, Carbs: 8g, Fiber: 4g, Fat: 7g, Cholesterol: 2mg, Sodium: 120mg, Potassium: 280mg.

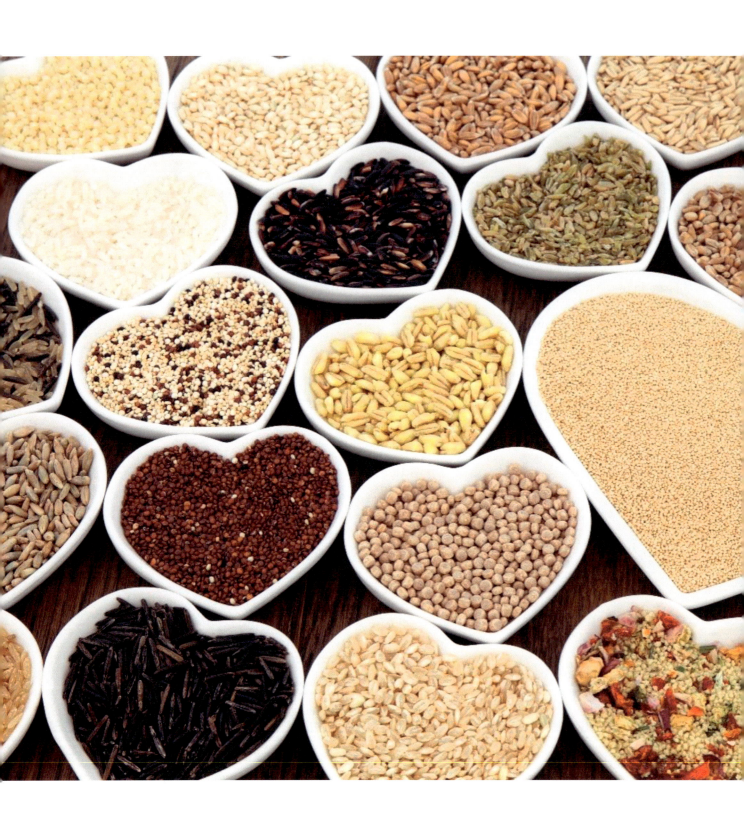

Recipe 117: Whole Wheat Pizza with Vegetables

Prep. time: 10 min | Cook time: 15 min | Serves: 3

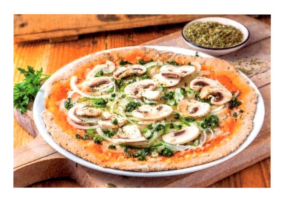

Ingredients:

1 package whole wheat pizza dough
1/2 cup reduced-sodium tomato sauce
1 cup part-skim mozzarella cheese, shredded
1 cup Mixed veggies - Capsicum, mushrooms, onions
1 teaspoon of dried basil
1 teaspoon of dried oregano
1 Tablespoon of Olive Oil.

Directions:

Preheat your oven to 450°F (230. Roll the dough out and spread with olive oil.
Spread tomato sauce, sprinkle the veggies, and grate cheese on top. Sprinkle some basil and oregano over the top.
Bake at 450°F for 12-15 minutes or until the crust is golden.

Nutritional Information (per serving, serves 4):

Calories: 300, Protein: 14g, Carbs: 40g, Fiber: 6g, Fat: 12g, Sodium: 280mg, Potassium: 300mg.

Recipe 118: Mushroom and Spinach Barley Risotto

Prep. time: 8 min | Cook time: 15 min | Serves: 2

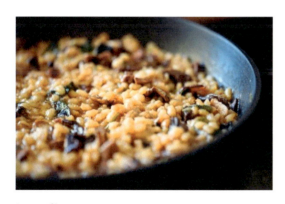

Ingredients:

1 cup pearl barley
4 cups low-sodium vegetable broth
1 cup mushrooms, sliced
2 cups fresh spinach
1 onion, chopped
2 cloves garlic, minced
2 tablespoons olive oil
1/4 cup Parmesan cheese
1 teaspoon of thyme.

Directions:

Heat the olive oil and sauté garlic and onion.
Add the barley and cook for 2 minutes.
Stir in the broth, a little at a time, and continue to cook until the barley is tender yet firm.
Add the mushrooms, spinach, thyme, and cheese; stir until the spinach wilts.
Serve and enjoy your risotto!

Nutritional information (per serving):

Calories: 199, Protein: 3g, Carbs: 7g, Fiber: 3g, Fat: 6g, Cholesterol: 20mg, Sodium: 55mg, Potassium: 150mg.

Recipe 119: Quinoa and Black Bean Bowl

Prep. time: 9 min | Cook time: 15 min | Serves: 3

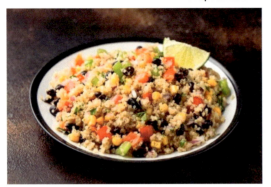

Directions:

Cook the quinoa in water according to the package instructions. Then, brown the onions, garlic, and bell pepper in olive oil.

Stir in beans, corn, cumin, and chili powder, and continue to heat through for about 5 minutes.

Top off the quinoa with the bean mixture and sprinkle with some fresh cilantro and a good squeeze of lime. Serve and enjoy your dish.

Nutritional Information (per serving):

Calories: 167, Protein: 6g, Carbs: 13g, Fiber: 2.3g, Fat: 5g, Cholesterol: 15mg, Sodium: 45mg, Potassium: 134mg.

Ingredients:

1 cup quinoa 2 cups water
1 can black beans, rinsed and drained
1 cup of corn
1 bell pepper, chopped
1 onion, chopped
2 Cloves Garlic, Minced
2 tablespoons olive oil
1 teaspoon cumin
1 tsp chili powder
1/4 cup Cilantro
Lime wedges to serve.

Recipe 120: Barley and Lentil Loaf

Prep. time: 7 min | Cook time: 75 min | Serves: 3

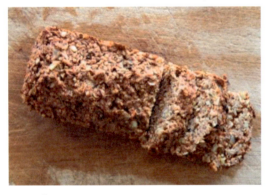

Directions:

Cook the barley and lentils in broth for 30-35 minutes until tender. Heat the oven to 375°F (190°C). Sweat the onions, garlic, carrots, and celery until soft. Combine the cooked barley and lentils with the sautéed vegetables, flaxseed, tomato paste, and spices.

Press the mixture into a loaf pan.

Bake for about 40-45 minutes until firm and golden on top.

Serve and enjoy your lentil loaf!

Nutritional information (per serving):

Calories: 146, Protein: 2.1g, Carbs: 8g, Fiber: 2.3g, Fat: 7g, Cholesterol: 30mg, Sodium: 70mg, Potassium: 220mg.

Ingredients:

1 cup pearl barley
1 cup Green lentils
4 cups low-sodium vegetable broth
1 onion, chopped
2 cloves of garlic, crushed
1 carrot, shredded
1 stalk of celery, minced
2 tablespoons ground flaxseed
2 tbsp tomato puree
1 teaspoon dried thyme
1 tsp smoked paprika
Salt and pepper to taste.

Recipe 121: Couscous and barley with veggies

Prep. time: 8 min | Cook time: 20 min | Serves: 3-4

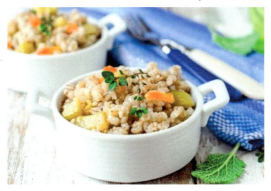

Ingredients:

1 Cup Pearl Barley, 1 cup whole wheat couscous, 3 cups Vegetable Broth
1 tablespoon olive oil, 1 medium onion, finely chopped, 2 carrots, chopped, 2 celery stalks, chopped, 2 cloves garlic, crushed
1 teaspoon cumin powder 1/2 teaspoon ground cori 1/4 cup fresh parsley, chopped
1/4 cup chopped fresh mint
Juice of 1 lemon, pepper to taste.

Directions:

Rinse barley and cook in a saucepan with 2 cups vegetable broth. Bring to a boil, reduce heat, cover, and simmer for 40 minutes until tender.

Combine whole wheat couscous in another bowl with 1 cup hot vegetable broth. Cover and let stand for 5 minutes. Heat olive oil in a large skillet over medium heat, sauté onion, carrots, and celery for 5-7 minutes until softened. Add garlic, cumin, and coriander, cooking for an additional minute.

Combine cooked barley, couscous, and sautéed vegetables. Mix in parsley, mint, and lemon juice. Season with black pepper.

Nutritional Information (per serving, serves 6):

Calories: 220, Protein: 7g, Carbs: 45g, Fiber: 8g, Fat: 3g, Cholesterol: 15mg, Sodium: 43mg, Potassium: 125mg.

Recipe 122: Millet and Roasted Vegetable Bowl

Prep. time: 12 min | Cook time: 45 min | Serves: 4

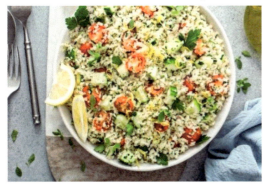

Ingredients:

1 cup millet
2 1/2 cups water
1 medium sweet potato, cubed
1 red bell pepper, sliced; 1 zucchini, sliced;
1 red onion, cut into wedges;
2 tablespoons olive oil;
1 teaspoon of dried rosemary
1 teaspoon thyme, dried,
2 cups kale, 1 tablespoon lemon juice,
1/4 cup sunflower.

Directions:

Preheat the oven to 400°F (200 C). Rinse the millet and combine it with water in a saucepan. Heat to boiling, reduce heat to simmering, and cook for 18-20 minutes or until all the water has evaporated. Toss the sweet potato, bell pepper, zucchini, and onion in 1 tablespoon olive oil with rosemary and thyme. Spread onto a prepared baking sheet and roast for 20 to 25 minutes.

Massage the kale with olive oil and lemon juice in a large bowl. Drop the cooked millet with a fork and divide it among serving bowls. Top with some roasted vegetables and massaged kale. Sprinkle some sunflower seeds on top before serving. Serve and enjoy your dish!

Nutritional information (per serving, serves 6):

Calories: 280, Protein: 14g, Carbs: 52g, Fiber: 13g, Fat: 3g, Sodium: 95mg, Potassium: 680mg.

Recipe 123: Butternut Squash and Sage Barley Risotto

Prep. time: 15 min | Cook time: 45 min | Serves: 6

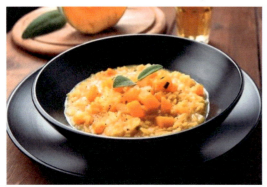

Ingredients:

1 small butternut squash, peeled
and diced (approximately three cups)
1 tablespoons of olive oil; 1 onion, finely
chopped; 2 cloves garlic, minced
1 cup pearl barley, rinsed
4 cups low-sodium vegetable broth
2 tablespoons of chopped clean sage
2 tablespoons of nutritional yeast
(optional). Salt and pepper to taste.

Directions:

Preheat the oven to 425°F (220°C). Toss the squash with half a tablespoon of olive oil and roast for 25 minutes until tender.

Meanwhile, in a large saucepan, heat the oil over medium heat. Sauté the onion until translucent. Add the garlic and barley, stirring for 1 minute. Add half a cup of broth at a time, stirring often and including extra as soon as absorbed, until the barley is tender (about forty minutes). Stir in the roasted squash, sage, and nutritional yeast. Season lightly with salt and pepper.

Serve and enjoy your risotto!

Nutritional Information (per serving):

Calories: 200, Protein: 5g, Carbs: 40g, Fiber: 8g, Fat: 3.5g, Cholesterol: 0mg, Sodium: 140mg, Potassium: 450mg.

Recipe 124: Heart-Healthy Freekeh with Roasted Eggplant

Prep. time: 18 min | Cook time: 40 min | Serves: 4

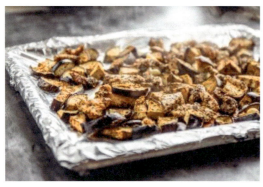

Ingredients:

1 large eggplant, cut into 1-inch cube; 2 tablespoons olive oil, divided
1/4 teaspoon salt, divided (or omit for lower sodium); 1/2 teaspoon black pepper, divided
1 cup of freekeh (cracked green wheat)
2 cups low-sodium vegetable broth or water;
1/4 cup pine nuts
1/4 cup fresh parsley, chopped
2 tablespoons lemon juice
2 cloves garlic, minced.

Directions:

Preheat oven to 400°F (200°C). Toss eggplant cubes with 1 tbsp olive oil, 1/8 tsp salt, and 1/4 tsp black pepper. Roast on a baking sheet for 25-30 minutes, stirring occasionally, until tender and browned.

In a saucepan, cook freekeh with vegetable broth or water: bring to a boil, reduce heat, and simmer for 20-25 minutes until tender and liquid is absorbed.

Toast pine nuts in a small skillet over medium heat for 2-3 minutes, stirring frequently.

In a large bowl, combine cooked freekeh, roasted eggplant, toasted pine nuts, parsley, lemon juice, minced garlic, remaining 1 tbsp olive oil, 1/8 tsp salt, and 1/4 tsp black pepper. Toss gently. Serve warm or at room temperature.

Nutritional information (per serving):

Calories: 310, Protein: 10g, Carbs: 30g, Fiber: 8g, Fat: 18g, Cholesterol: 0mg, Sodium: 580mg, Potassium: 550mg.

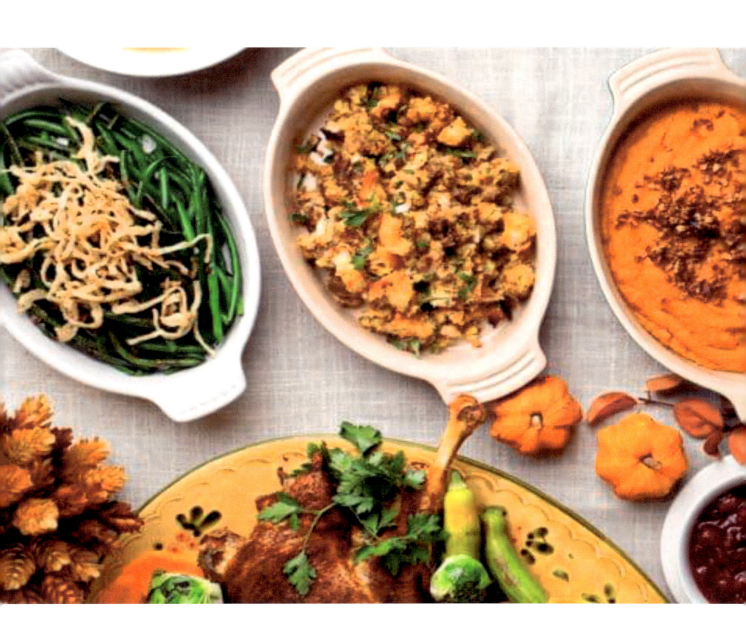

Recipe 125: Spinach Falafel

Prep. time: 10 min | Cook time: 25 min | Serves: 3-4

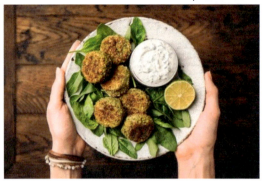

Ingredients:

1 cup of water
6 tbsp of extra virgin olive oil
1 chopped onion
1 Pound of spinach, chopped, blanched and well drained
1 cup of Greek yogurt
2 tablespoons of almond flour
6 tablespoons of shelled and peeled pistachios
3 tablespoons of chopped fresh cilantro
Oregano and ground black pepper.

Directions:

Set the oven to 200°C (400°F). In a medium bowl, dissolve the falafel mix in water and let stand for 15 minutes, then shape into eight falafels. Heat 2 tbsp oil in a large, non-stick skillet over moderate heat. Sauté the onion for 1 minute until soft. Add spinach, salt, and pepper; cook for 2 minutes, stirring constantly. Combine yogurt with flour and pour over the spinach. Transfer to an unbuttered baking dish. Heat the remaining oil in the skillet and brown the falafels for 2-3 minutes on each side. Place falafels on the spinach. Bake, uncovered, for 15-20 minutes until bubbling. Top with pistachios and coriander. Serve and enjoy! Serve and enjoy your dish!

Nutritional information (per serving, serves 6):

Calories: 230, Protein: 6g, Carbs: 43g, Fiber: 2g, Fat: 7g, Cholesterol: 25mg, Sodium: 68mg, Potassium: 230mg.

Recipe 126: Cauliflower sticks

Prep. time: 12min | Cook time: 40min | Serves: 6

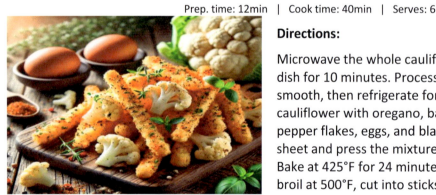

Ingredients:

1 Medium cauliflower head
½ Tablespoon of oregano
1 Tablespoon of basil
1 Tablespoon of onion powder
½ Teaspoon of red pepper flakes
2 Large eggs
1 Pinch of ground black pepper.

Directions:

Microwave the whole cauliflower head in a heat-proof dish for 10 minutes. Process it in a food processor until smooth, then refrigerate for 10 minutes. Mix the cauliflower with oregano, basil, onion powder, red pepper flakes, eggs, and black pepper. Grease a baking sheet and press the mixture onto it, about ½ inch thick. Bake at 425°F for 24 minutes. Remove, set the oven to broil at 500°F, cut into sticks, flip, and broil for 15 minutes until golden and crispy. Serve and enjoy!

Nutritional Information (per serving, serves 6):

Calories: 280, Protein: 14g, Carbs: 52g, Fiber: 13g, Fat: 3g, Sodium: 95mg, Potassium: 680mg.

Recipe 127: Pine Nut Pesto

Prep. time: 10 min | Cook time: 20 min | Serves: 4

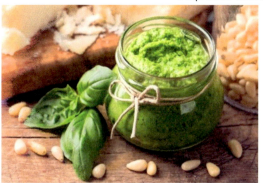

Ingredients:

2 Cups basil, fresh and finely chopped
2 Cloves garlic, finely chopped
½ Cup pine nuts, toasted
½ Cup extra virgin olive oil
1 ¼ tsp lemon juice, freshly squeezed
1 Pinch oregano.

Directions:

Place the basil, pine nuts, lemon juice, and garlic in a food processor and pulse until your ingredients are finely chopped. Gradually add the olive oil and process until your ingredients are very- combined. Season with the oregano and pepper. Transfer the mixture to a jar and cover with a small amount of olive oil. Store the pesto in the refrigerator or use it right away. Enjoy!

Nutritional information (per serving, serves 6):

Calories: 223, Protein: 2g, Carbs: 12g, Fiber: 2.1g, Fat: 4g, Cholesterol: 30mg, Sodium: 80mg, Potassium: 250mg.

Recipe 128: Roasted Savoy Cabbage with Orange Vinaigrette

Prep. time: 15 min | Cook time: 25 min | Serves: 4

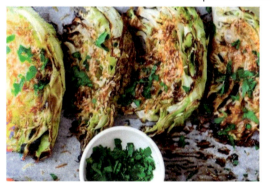

Ingredients:

1 small head of savoy cabbage
(about 1 pound), cut into wedges
2 tablespoons olive oil
1/4 teaspoon salt
1/4 teaspoon black pepper
1/4 cup fresh orange juice
2 tablespoons apple cider vinegar
1 tablespoon Dijon mustard
1 teaspoon of maple syrup
2 tablespoons olive oil (for the vinaigrette)
2 tablespoons chopped fresh parsley.

Directions:

Toss the savoy cabbage wedges in a large bowl with 2 tablespoons of olive oil, salt, and black pepper until well coated. Arrange the cabbage wedges in a single layer on a baking sheet. Roast for 20-25 minutes until the cabbage is tender and lightly charred, flipping halfway through.
While the cabbage is roasting, prepare the vinaigrette by whisking together the orange juice, apple cider vinegar, Dijon mustard, honey, and 2 tablespoons of olive oil in a small bowl. Remove the roasted cabbage from the oven and transfer to a serving platter.
Drizzle the orange vinaigrette over the roasted cabbage and sprinkle with chopped fresh parsley.
Serve warm or at room temperature.

Nutritional information (per serving):

Calories: 180, Protein: 2g, Carbs: 12g, Fiber: 4g, Fat: 14g, Cholesterol: 0mg, Sodium: 160mg, Potassium: 320mg.

Recipe 129: Easy heart, healthy Guacamole

Prep. time: 15min | Cook time: 15 min | Serves: 4

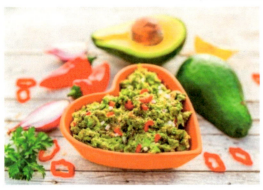

Ingredients:

3 ripe avocados; 1/4 cup diced red onion
2 tablespoons fresh lime juice
1 Roma tomato, diced;
2 tablespoons chopped fresh cilantro;
1 clove garlic, minced;
1/4 teaspoon ground cumin
1/8 teaspoon cayenne pepper (optional)
1/4 teaspoon salt.

Directions:

Cut avocados in half, remove pits, and scoop flesh into a bowl. Add diced red onion, lime juice, tomato, cilantro, minced garlic, cumin, and cayenne pepper (if using). Mash to desired consistency. Fold in salt gently. Adjust seasoning if needed.

Serve immediately with fresh vegetables or whole-grain tortilla chips.

Nutritional Information (per serving):

Calories: 230, Protein: 3g, Carbs: 13g, Fiber: 8g, Fat: 20g, Cholesterol: 0mg, Sodium: 120mg, Potassium: 690m.

Recipe 130: Mediterranean Grilled Vegetable Skewers

Prep. time: 15min | Cook time: 15 min | Serves: 4

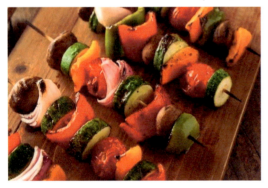

Ingredients:

2 zucchinis, sliced into 1-inch
2 yellow squashes, sliced into 1-inch pieces;
1 red onion, cut into 1-inch chunks
1 red bell pepper, cut into 1-inch pieces
1 yellow bell pepper, cut into 1-inch pieces
12 cherry tomatoes;
1/4 cup of olive oil
2 t balsamic vinegar;
2 cloves garlic, minced
1 teaspoon dry oregano;
1/2 teaspoon dried basil.
Salt pepper to taste.

Directions:

Cut avocados in half, remove pits, and scoop flesh into a bowl. Add diced red onion, lime juice, tomato, cilantro, minced garlic, cumin, and cayenne pepper (if using). Mash to desired consistency. Fold in salt gently. Adjust seasoning if needed.

Serve immediately with fresh vegetables or whole-grain tortilla chips.

Nutritional Information (per serving):

Calories: 230, Protein: 3g, Carbs: 13g, Fiber: 8g, Fat: 20g, Cholesterol: 0mg, Sodium: 120mg, Potassium: 690m.

Recipe 131: Lentil and Mushroom Stuffed Bell Peppers

Prep. time: 20 min | Cook time: 40 min | Serves: 6

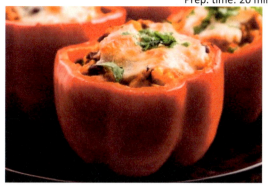

Ingredients:

6 bell peppers with the tops eliminated and seeded; 1 cup of brown lentils, rinsed;
2 cups water; 1 tablespoon of olive oil
1 onion, diced;
2 cloves garlic, minced
8 ounces of mushrooms, chopped
1 teaspoon of dried thyme;
1 tablespoon of tomato paste;
1/4 cup of chopped fresh parsley.
Salt and pepper to taste.

Directions:

Preheat oven to 375°F (190°C).
Cook lentils in water until smooth, approximately 20 minutes. Drain any extra water. In a skillet, heat oil over medium heat. Sauté onion till translucent. Add garlic and mushrooms, cooking until mushrooms release their moisture. Stir in cooked lentils, thyme, tomato paste, salt, and pepper. Fill bell peppers with the lentil mixture in a baking dish.
Cover with foil and bake for 30-35 minutes until peppers are soft. Sprinkle with parsley before serving. Serve and enjoy your dish!

Nutritional Information (per serving):

Calories: 170, Protein: 9g, Carbs: 28g, Fiber: 11g, Fat: 3.5g, Cholesterol: 0mg, Sodium: 95mg, Potassium: 680mg

Recipe 132: Stuffed Sweet Potatoes

Prep. time: 15 min | Cook time: 60 min | Serves: 6

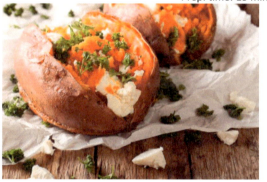

Ingredients:

6 medium sweet potatoes;
1/2 cup low-fat Greek yogurt;
1/2 cup low-fat feta cheese, crumbled; 2 green onions, thinly sliced;
1/2 cup of diced tomatoes
1/2 cup diced cucumbers;
1/four cup chopped parsley;
1/4 cup chopped fresh dill;
1 tablespoon of olive oil;
1 tablespoon of lemon juice and 1 teaspoon of dried oregano.
Salt and pepper to taste. Corn kernels.

Directions:

Preheat your oven to 400°F (200°C). Wash and prick the sweet potatoes with a fork. Bake them directly on the oven rack for 45-60 minutes until tender. While baking, mix Greek yogurt with feta cheese. In another bowl, combine tomatoes, cucumbers, parsley, dill, olive oil, lemon juice, and oregano, season with salt and pepper. Once the potatoes are done, let them cool briefly, then cut a slit lengthwise and fluff the insides with a fork. Fill each potato with the yogurt-feta mixture and top with the tomato-cucumber mix and green onions. Add any additional toppings as desired.
Serve and enjoy your side dish!

Nutritional Information (per serving):

Calories: 189, Protein: 9g, Carbs: 28g, Fiber: 4g, Fat: 5g, Saturated Fat: 2g, Cholesterol: 10mg, Sodium: 200mg, Potassium: 500mg.

Recipe 133: Herb-Roasted Sweet Potatoes

Prep. time: 10 min | Cook time: 30 min | Serves: 2

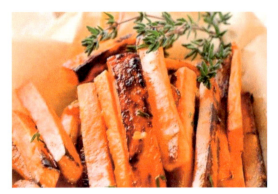

Directions:

Preheat oven to 425°F. Toss sweet potatoes with oil and herbs.
Roast for 25-30 minutes, turning halfway through.
Serve and enjoy your dish!

Nutritional information (per serving, serves 4):

Calories: 100 Protein: 1g Carbs: 18g Fiber: 3g Fat: 3g
Sodium: 35mg Potassium: 350mg.

Ingredients:

2 medium sweet potatoes, cubed
1 tablespoon of olive oil
1 teaspoon of dried rosemary
1 teaspoon of dried thyme
1/4 teaspoon of ground black pepper.

Recipe 134: Lemom herb Couscous

Prep time: 18 min | Cook time: 10 min | Serves: 3

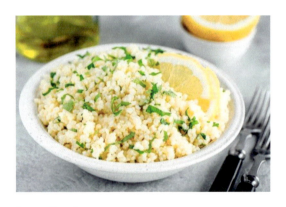

Directions:

Bring the broth to a boil, then add in the couscous
Remove from the heat and cover.
Let stand for about 5 minutes, then fluff with the help of a fork.
Stir in the lemon juice, herbs, the almonds, and the oil.
Serve and enjoy your dish!

Nutritional information (per serving, serves 4):

Calories: 200, Protein: 6g, Carbs: 30g, Fiber: 4g, Fat: 7g,
Sodium: 15mg, Potassium: 180mg.

Ingredients:

1 cup of whole wheat couscous
1 and 1/4 cups of low-sodium vegetable broth
2 tablespoons of lemon juice
1/4 cup of chopped fresh herbs (parsley, mint, cilantro)
1/4 cup of slivered almonds, toasted
1 tablespoon of olive oil.

CHAPTER 7: DESSERTS WITH BENEFITS

7.1. SWEET, SAFE INDULGENCE

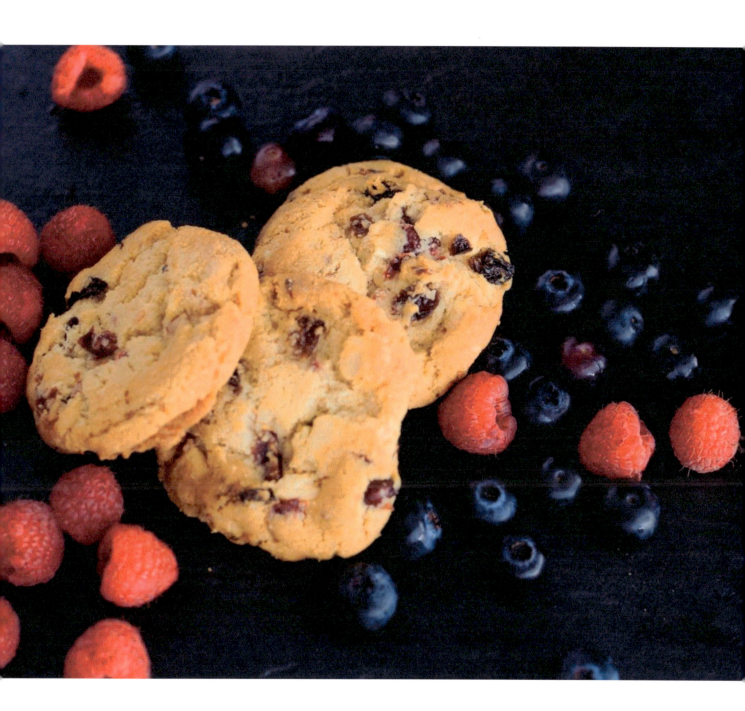

Recipe 135: Oatmeal Cookies

Prep time: 10min | Cook time: 12 min | Serves: 8

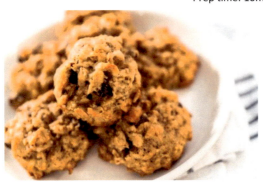

Ingredients:

1 cup rolled oats
1/2 cup almond flour
1/4 cup unsweetened applesauce
1/4 cup unsweetened almond milk
1/4 cup ripe banana, mashed
1 teaspoon vanilla extract
1/2 teaspoon ground cinnamon
1/4 teaspoon baking powder
A pinch of salt.

Directions:

Prepare oven to 350°F (175°C). Line a cookie sheet with parchment paper. In a bowl, mix all the ingredients until well combined. With a scoop, shape the dough into cookies on the prepared baking sheet. Bake until golden, 12-15 minutes. Let cool then ready to serve.
Serve and enjoy your dessert!

Nutritional information (per cookie):

Calories: 60, Protein: 2g, Carbs: 8g, Fiber: 2g, Fat: 3g, Cholesterol: 0mg, Sodium: 40mg, Potassium: 120mg.

Recipe 136: Chocolate-Fudge Pudding Cake

Prep. time: 10min | Cook time: 25-30min | Serves: 8

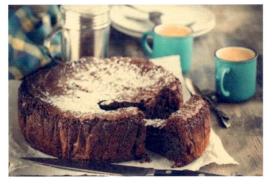

Ingredients:

1 cup cocoa powder
1/2 cup blanched almond flour
1 teaspoon baking powder
1/4 teaspoon salt
1 cup unsweetened almond milk
1/2 cup ripe mashed banana
1 teaspoon vanilla extract
1/4 cup unsweetened applesauce.

Directions:

Preheat oven to 350°F (175°C). Butter an 8-inch baking dish.
Gradually blend in a bowl: cocoa powder, almond flour, baking powder, and salt.
Mix almond milk, mashed banana, vanilla, and applesauce in another bowl.
Combine the wet ingredients into the dry ones and mix to combine.
Pour the batter into the prepared baking dish.
Place the cake in the oven and bake for about 25-30 minutes, checking the center with a toothpick for doneness.
Allow it to stand and cool down before serving.
Serve and enjoy your dessert!

Nutritional information (per serving):

Calories: 120, Protein: 4g, Carbs: 16g, Fiber: 5g, Fat: 5g, Cholesterol: 0mg, Sodium: 120mg, Potassium: 300mg.

Recipe 137: Healthy Cookies

Prep. time: 10 min | Cook time: 12-15 min | Serves: 12

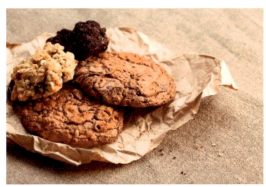

Ingredients:

1 1/2 cups almond flour
1/2 cup unsweetened applesauce
1/4 cup unsweetened almond milk
1 teaspoon vanilla extract
1/2 teaspoon baking powder
1/4 teaspoon salt.

Directions:

Preheat the oven to 350°F (175°C). Line the baking sheet with parchment paper.
Mix the almond flour, applesauce, almond milk, vanilla, baking powder, and salt.
Shape the dough into cookies using an ice cream scoop and place on the lined baking sheet.
Bake for about 12-15 minutes or until lightly browned.
Allow to cool then serve.
Serve and enjoy your dessert!

Nutritional information (per cookie):

Calories: 80, Protein: 3g, Carbs: 6g, Fiber: 2g, Fat: 6g, Cholesterol: 0mg, Sodium: 60mg, Potassium: 90mg.

Recipe 138: Meringues

Prep. time: 10 min | Cook time: 60 min | Serves: 6

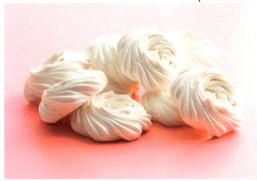

Ingredients:

4 egg whites
1/4 teaspoon cream of tartar
1/4 cup unsweetened applesauce
1 teaspoon vanilla extract.

Directions:

Preheat the oven to 225°F (105°C). Line a baking sheet with parchment paper.
Beat the egg whites in a mixing bowl with an electric mixer until frothy.
Add the cream of tartar and continue whipping until soft peaks form.
Gradually beat in the applesauce and vanilla extract until stiff, shiny peaks form.
Pipe or spoon the meringue onto the prepared baking sheet.
Bake for 1 hour in a preheated 200°F oven, then turn off the oven and set it for 1 hour. Remove the bread from the oven and let it cool completely before serving.

Nutritional information (per meringue):

Calories: 20, Protein: 2g, Carbs: 2g, Fiber: 0g, Fat: 0g, Cholesterol: 0mg, Sodium: 25mg, Potassium: 30mg.

Recipe 139: Apple Crisp

Prep. time: 15min | Cook time: 30-35 min | Serves: 8

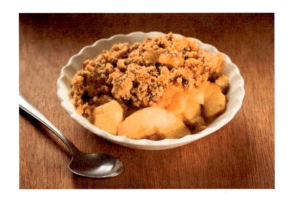

Ingredients:

4 apples, peeled, cored, and sliced
1 teaspoon of cinnamon
1/2 teaspoon grated nutmeg
1 cup rolled oats
1/2 cup almond flour
1/4 cup unsweetened applesauce
2 tablespoons coconut oil, melted.

Directions:

Preheat your oven to about 350 degrees F (175 degrees C). Grease an 8-inch. Spread the sliced apples on the base of a baking dish and sprinkle the cinnamon and nutmeg over the apples.

Mix the rolled oats, almond flour, applesauce, and melted coconut oil in a separate bowl. Crumble the oat mix over the apples. Place this dish in the oven and bake for 30-35 minutes until the topping is golden brown and the apples are slightly tender. Let it cool before serving.

Nutritional information (per serving):

Calories: 210, Protein: 4g, Carbs: 30g, Fiber: 6g, Fat: 9g, Cholesterol: 0mg, Sodium: 30mg, Potassium: 250mg.

Recipe 140: Cinnamon-Raisin Oatmeal Cookies

Prep. time: 10min | Cook time: 12-15 min | Serves: 12

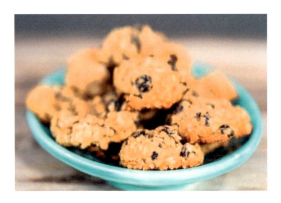

Ingredients:

1 cup old-fashioned rolled oats
1/2 cup almond meal
1/4 cup unsweetened applesauce
1/4 cup mashed ripe banana
1 teaspoon vanilla extract
1 teaspoon ground cinnamon
1/4 teaspoon baking powder
1/4 teaspoon salt
1/4 cup raisins.

Directions:

Preheat oven to 350°F. Cover a baking sheet with parchment paper.
Combine all ingredients except the raisins in a bowl until all mixed in.
Add the raisins and fold in.
Scoop the dough and shape it into cookies on the prepared baking sheet.
Bake for 12-15 minutes or until lightly brown.
Allow to cool and then serve.
Enjoy your dessert!

Nutritional information (per cookie): Calories:

81, Protein: 3g, Carbs: 11g, Fiber: 1.9g, Fat: 4g, Cholesterol: 0mg, Sodium: 30mg, Potassium: 140mg.

7.2. LOW-FAT BAKING SECRETS

While conventional baking frequently relies on butter, sugar, and unhealthy fats, there are smart strategies you may adapt to craft scrumptious and nutritious heart-healthy, low-sodium baked goods ideal for your daily lifestyle. One key strategy is to include substitutions. Swap out butter for healthier alternatives like applesauce, mashed banana, or unsweetened fruit puree. These alternatives add moisture and sweetness without the saturated fat in butter. When it comes to sugar, discover herbal sweeteners like honey or maple syrup; however, bear in mind to apply them moderately. You can even try decreasing the general quantity of sugar in recipes, as your taste buds will step by step adjust to a much less candy palate. Here are some other techniques for Low-Fat Baking Secrets

Use Citrus Zest: Lemon, lime, and orange zest can brighten the flavor profile of each sweet and savory baked object.

Baking Soda (Sodium Bicarbonate): When lowering baking soda, you could use potassium bicarbonate and a bit of acid (like lemon juice or vinegar) to preserve the leavening impact.

Baking Powder: Choose sodium-unfastened baking powder, which is commercially available and works just as well as the conventional model.

Alternative Ingredients:

Unsalted Butter: Always pick out unsalted butter to manage over the sodium ingredients.

Low-Sodium Broth or Stock: Replace regular broth with low-sodium or self-made versions of savory baked ingredients like bread or biscuits.

Homemade ingredients: Make your very own ketchup, mustard, and different condiments to keep away from the high sodium degrees observed in save-sold types.

Dough and Batter Modifications:

Yeast Bread: Reduce the salt through half and add a piece natural sweetener to catch up on the flavor loss.

Flavor Enhancers:

Umami-Rich Ingredients: Incorporate low-sodium, umami-rich meals like mushrooms, tomatoes, and seaweeds to improve the savory taste without adding salt.

Sweet and Savory Balance: For sweet baked items, use natural sweeteners like honey, maple syrup, or fruit purees, which may add complexity and decrease the need for salt.

Adjusting Baking Methods

Use of Egg Whites: Substitute whole eggs with egg whites or egg substitutes to reduce fat and cholesterol.

Incorporating Air: Techniques like whipping egg whites to stiff peaks and folding them into the batter can introduce air and lightness, compensating for fat loss.

Watch Baking Time: Low-fat cookies may bake faster, so keep an eye on them to prevent drying out.

Whole Grains: Use whole wheat flour or oats to increase fiber and nutrients while maintaining the structure.

Note:

Low-fat baking doesn't mean sacrificing flavor or enjoyment. With the correct substitutions, techniques, and a bit of creativity, you can produce delicious, healthier baked goods. Remember, the goal is to create a balance that maintains the integrity of the baked item while reducing the fat content. And don't be afraid to test and locate what works for you. With some creativity and these available tips, you can revel in delicious and heart-healthy baked items that can be a great addition to any weight loss plan.

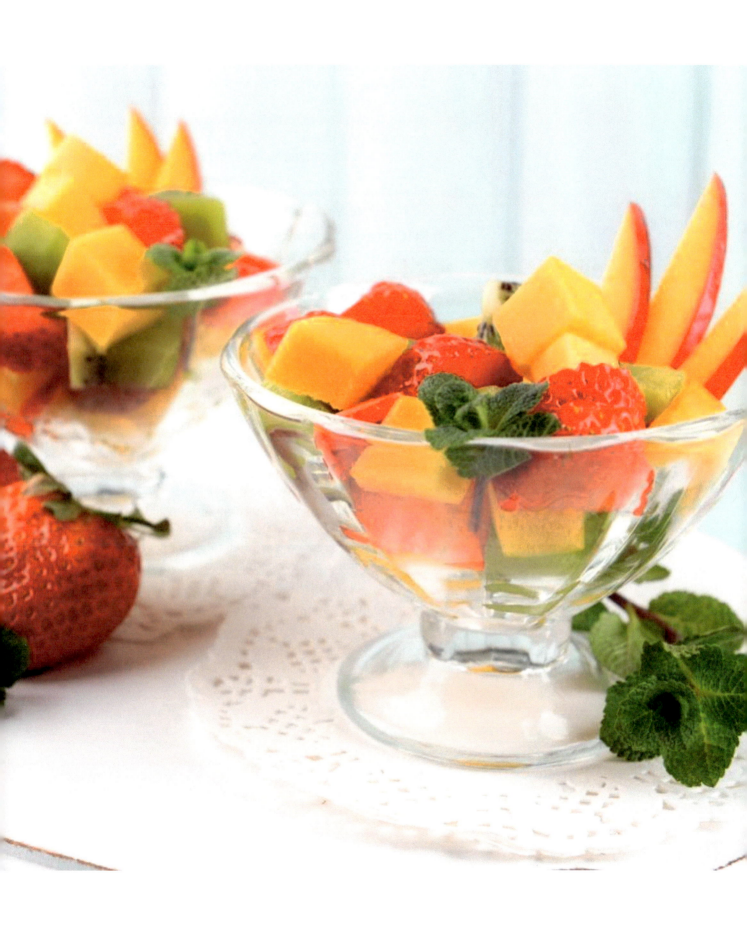

Recipe 141: Baked Apple Chips

Prep. time: 10 min | Cook time: 2 hours | Serves: 3-4

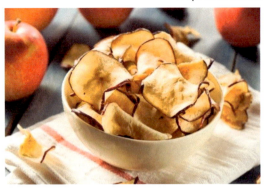

Ingredients:

2 large apples, sliced thin
1 teaspoon ground cinnamon
1 tablespoon fresh lemon juice.

Directions:

Preheat the oven to 200°F (93°C).
Sprinkle the apple slices with the cinnamon and lemon juice.
Lay the apple slices in a single layer on a parchment paper-covered baking sheet.
Bake for 2 hours, turning halfway through, or until dry and crisp.
Allow to cool completely before serving.
Serve and enjoy your dessert!

Nutritional Information (per serving):

Calories 60, 0g Protein, 16g Carbs, 3g Fiber, 0g Fat, 0mg Cholesterol, 0mg Sodium, 120mg Potassium.

Recipe 142: Strawberry-Banana Ice Cream

Prep. time: 10 min | Cook time: 2 Hours | Serves: 4

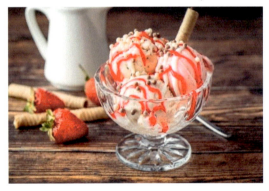

Ingredients:

2 cups frozen strawberries
2 ripe bananas, frozen
1/4 cup unsweetened almond milk
1 teaspoon vanilla extract.

Directions:

Purée strawberries, bananas, almond milk, and vanilla extract in a food processor or blender.
Blend until your ingredients become smooth and creamy, scraping down the sides of the blender.
Transfer the ice cream to a freezer-safe container and freeze for 2 hours before serving.
Serve and enjoy your dessert!

Nutrition Information (per serving):

Calories: 100, Protein: 2g, Carbs: 24g, Fiber: 4g, Fat: 1g, Cholesterol: 0mg, Sodium: 10mg, Potassium: 470mg.

Recipe 143: Grilled Peaches with Cinnamon Coconut Cream

Prep. time: 10 min | Cook time: 8 min | Serves: 4

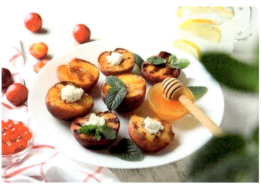

Ingredients:

4 ripe peaches, halved and pitted
1 can full-fat coconut milk, refrigerated
1 teaspoon vanilla extract
1 teaspoon cinnamon
1/4 teaspoon ground cardamom (optional).

Directions:

Open the can of coconut milk from the refrigerator and spoon the thickened coconut cream into a bowl, reserving the liquid for another use.
Add the vanilla, cinnamon, and cardamom to the coconut cream and whip until stiff peaks form. Grill the peach halves on medium heat for 3-4 minutes on each side until lightly charred. Divide the broiled peaches into plates and sprinkle each half with a dollop of cinnamon coconut cream.

Nutrition Information:

Calories: 86, Protein: 4g, Carbs: 8g, Fiber: 2.5g, Fat: 9.8g, Cholesterol: 0mg, Sodium: 30mg, Potassium: 146mg.

Recipe 144: Chocolate-dipped Strawberry Bites

Prep. time: 20 min | Cook time: 10 min | Serves: 5 (24 strawberries)

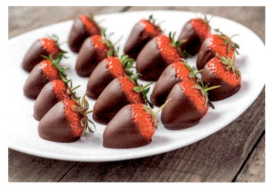

Ingredients:

16 ounces fresh strawberries
1/2 cup coconut, melted
1/4 cup unsweetened cocoa
1 tablespoon unsweetened almond milk
1/4 teaspoon vanilla extract.

Directions:

Rinse strawberries and pat them very dry. Leave them with stems. Combine the cocoa powder, vanilla, and almond milk with the coconut butter in a medium bowl. Dip the stem of each strawberry in chocolate so that approximately 3/4 of the way up the fruit is covered. Lay the dipped strawberries on a baking sheet lined with parchment paper. Let chill them in the refrigerator for 30 minutes or until they have set.

Nutrition Information (per 4 strawberries):

Calories: 110, Protein: 2g, Carbs: 7g, Fiber: 3g, Fat: 9g, Cholesterol: 0mg, Sodium: 0mg, Potassium: 160mg.

Recipe 145: Mint and Lime Fruit Salad

Prep. time: 5 min | Cook time: 15 min | Serves: 3

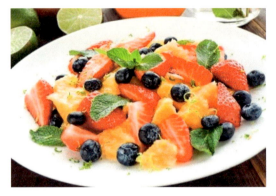

Directions:

In a large bowl, combine the fruits.
In a small bowl, whisk the lime juice and the honey.
Toss the fruits with the dressing and the mint.
Serve and enjoy your fruit salad!

Nutritional information (per serving):

Calories: 90, Protein: 1g, Carbohydrates: 23g, Fiber: 3g, Sugars: 19g, Fat: 0g, Cholesterol: 0mg, Sodium: 5mg, Potassium: 220mg.

Ingredients:

4 cups mixed fruit chunks (melon, berries, grapes, etc.)
2 tablespoons lime juice
2 tablespoons honey
1/4 cup fresh mint, chopped.

Recipe 146: Fruit Kabobs

Prep. time: 5 min | Cook time: 5 min | Serves: 2

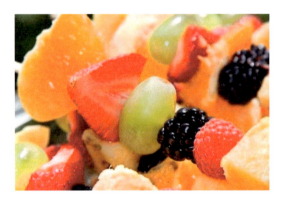

Directions:

Thread the fruit onto skewers.
Mix the oil with the honey, cinnamon, and lime juice.
Brush the mixture over the fruit.
Grill for about 2 to 3 minutes per side.
Serve and enjoy your fruit Kabobs!

Nutritional information (per serving, serves 4):

Calories: 100, Protein: 1g, Carbs: 22g, Fiber: 2g, Fat: 3g, Sodium: 1mg, Potassium.

Ingredients:

2 cups of mixed fruit chunks (pineapple, blueberries, peaches, plums)
1 tablespoon of olive oil
1 tablespoon of honey
1 teaspoon of cinnamon
The Juice of 1 lime.

Recipe 147: Spiced Baked Plums

Prep. time: 5 min | Cook time: 25 min | Serves: 2

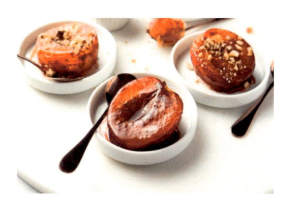

Ingredients:

4 plums, halved and pitted
2 tablespoons of honey
1 teaspoon of ground cinnamon
1/4 teaspoon of ground nutmeg
1/4 cup chopped pecans.

Directions:

Preheat your oven to 375°F.
Place the plums cut side up in a baking dish.
Drizzle with honey and sprinkle with cinnamon, nutmeg, and pecans.
Bake for about 20-25 minutes until tender.
Serve and enjoy your dessert!

Nutritional Information (per serving, serves 4):

Calories: 130, Protein: 1g, Carbs: 20g, Fiber: 3g, Fat: 5g, Sodium: 1mg, Potassium: 190mg.

Recipe 148: Plum and Almond Tart

Prep. time: 10 min | Cook time: 25 min | Serves: 4

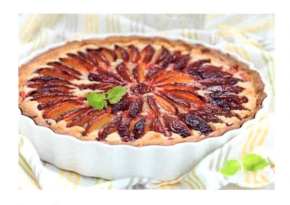

Ingredients:

6 ripe plums, halved and pitted
1 cup almond flour
2 tablespoons of olive oil
2 tablespoons of honey
1 egg
1/2 teaspoon of almond extract
1/4 cup sliced almonds.

Directions:

Preheat your oven to 375°F.
Mix the almond flour, oil, 1 tbsp honey, egg, and almond extract.
Press your mixture right into a tart pan.
Arrange the plums on the pinnacle and drizzle them with honey.
Sprinkle with the sliced almonds.
Bake for about 25 minutes until golden
Serve and enjoy your dessert!

Nutritional Information (per serving, serves 6):

Calories: 220, Protein: 7g, Carbs: 20g, Fiber: 4g, Fat: 15g, Sodium: 10mg, Potassium: 220mg.

Recipe 149: Frozen Banana Pops

Prep. time: 10 min | Cook time: 240 min | Serves: 4

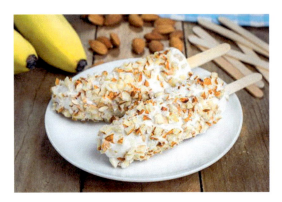

Directions:

Cut the bananas in half, then insert them into the popsicle sticks.
Mix the yogurt and the honey.
Dip the bananas in the yogurt mixture, then roll in the nuts and coconut.
Freeze for a minimum of 2 hours.
Serve and enjoy your dessert!

Nutritional Information (per serving):

Calories: 120, Protein: 3g, Carbs: 18g, Fiber: 2g, Fat: 5g, Sodium: 5mg, Potassium: 240mg.

Ingredients:

4 ripe bananas
½ cup Greek yogurt
2 tablespoons of honey
1/4 cup chopped nuts (almonds, peanuts, or walnuts)
1/4 cup unsweetened shredded coconut.

Recipe 150: Grapefruit Brûlée

Prep. time: 5 min | Cook time: 25 min | Serves: 3

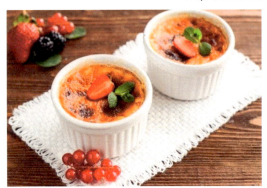

Directions:

Cut the grapefruits into halves
Remove the seeds of the grapefruit
Mix the honey and vanilla and brush over the grapefruit halves.
Broil for about 2-3 minutes till the grapefruits are caramelized.
Serve with a dollop of Greek yogurt.
Serve and enjoy your dessert!

Nutritional Information (per serving):

Calories: 90, Protein: 3g, Carbs: 20g, Fiber: 2g, Fat: 0g, Sodium: 10mg, Potassium.

Ingredients:

2 cups of grapefruits
2 tablespoons of honey
¼ teaspoon of vanilla extract
¼ cup of Greek yogurt.

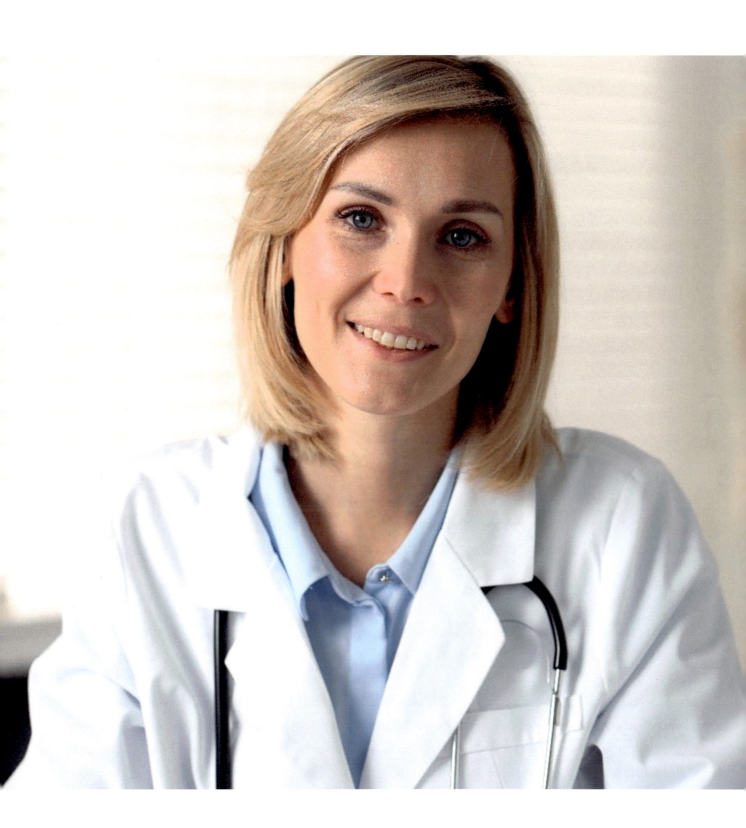

8.1 TIPS FROM NUTRITIONISTS AND CARDIOLOGISTS

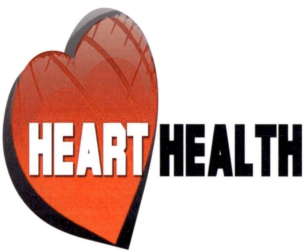

In the process of keeping your cardiovascular system strong, maintaining a heart-healthy diet is the single most potent tool for reducing your risk of heart disease. This doesn't mean drastic changes or deprivation. It's about adding more of the good stuff and pulling back a little on a few things. The best example was a large study published in the *New England Journal of Medicine*, which followed over 15,000 adults for almost twenty years. The key takeaway was that the most adherent to a heart-healthy diet, rich in fruits, vegetables, whole grains, healthy fats from olive oil, and nuts, had a 25% lower risk of developing cardiovascular disease than those who did not follow this eating pattern. Another review of 41 studies with over 800,000 participants reported that for a 2-serving per day increase in whole grains, there was an 8% lower risk of heart disease. But replacing red meat with plant-based proteins like beans and lentils for even just eight weeks in a clinical trial at the Cleveland Clinic impacted beneficially on cholesterol numbers, amongst other factors associated with heart disease. Making small, sustainable changes towards an emphasis on nutrient-dense, minimally processed food and reducing foods high in saturated fat, sodium, and added sugar can make significant strides in support of long-term heart health. Here are some essential tips straight from the expertise of nutritionists and cardiologists to steer you toward a heart-loving way of eating:

A Diet rich in fiber:

Nutritionists recommend whole grain foods, fruits, vegetables, and legumes to ensure the heart is well cared for. One of the healthiest strategies for heart care is consuming fiber-rich food. Fiber is known to help individuals lower their blood fats and check their blood sugar. An applicable example is white bread, which can be swapped with whole-grain bread. If possible, you can add brown rice, quinoa, and oats to your daily diet, as they are excellent sources of fiber. Furthermore, all these food groups provide essential vitamins, minerals, and antioxidants, promoting heart health in the diet. Various colored fruits and vegetables offer multiple more effective nutrients when they work together to provide health benefits. For example, include a few lentils in your favorite soups and salads to boost the fiber and protein in a nourishing and filling meal. Avoid Saturated and Trans Fats. Cardiologists recommend minimizing saturated fat consumption in red meat, butter, and full-fat dairy products. Consuming too much-saturated fat elevates LDL (bad) cholesterol levels and increases the chance of getting heart disease. Instead, they advise one to take lean meat and low-fat dairy and get most of the fat from the plant. Red meat should not be consumed in large quantities due to high saturated fats, specifically ribeye and brisket, with very high fat content. Avoid them and opt for slimmer red meat, such as sirloin, round steak, or skinless poultry and fish. Butter and full-fat dairy products also have high levels of saturated fats. Some of the healthier alternatives include olive oil, avocado, or low-fat dairy products. Nuts and seeds other than almonds and walnuts also include chia seeds, an excellent source of unsaturated fats with an advantage to the heart.

Include more omega-3 fatty acids: Nutritionists worldwide suggest including oily fish containing omega-3 fatty acids in one's diet as it is perfect for one's heart. These healthy fats can lower the amount of triglycerides and the amount of inflammation, thus generally benefiting heart health. A superb source of omega-3 fatty acids is salmon. Grill or bake the fish to create a delicious, healthy addition to the diet each week. Other exceptional options are mackerel and sardines, which are also offered in quite a range of dishes or, as a more convenient, canned rendition. Aim to get your omega-3 fatty acids from a high-quality fish oil supplement if you're not consuming at least two fish meals per week. The appropriate dose will vary based on your profile and should be prescribed by a physician or dietitian. Opt for Lean Sources of Protein Cardiologists prefer skinless poultry, fish, tofu, and legumes to fatty cuts of beef and processed meats like bacon and sausage. Lean proteins are essential to having a healthy heart. They contain a smaller proportion of saturated fats than some of the high-fat percentage cuts of meat, as well as processed meats. Skinless chicken breast and turkey breast are excellent sources of lean proteins that can be prepared in numerous ways, including baking, grilling, or sautéing with the use of heart-healthy oil. The sources include good lean protein as well as omega-3 from fish. Other plant-based proteins to be sourced from tofu and legumes like lentils, chickpeas, and black beans are naturally low in saturated fats but high in fiber. These all can be made into tasty salads or included in stir-fries, or they can be used as meat in something like chili or a vegetable patty.

Increase intake of fruits and vegetables: Nutritionists have always recommended making half of your plate full of different colors of fruits and vegetables in every meal. It gives you all the necessary vitamins, minerals, and antioxidants, and it also serves as a good source of fiber that can be pretty useful in considering heart health. Good examples are that when you eat spinach and kale, you take lots of folate, vitamin K, and magnesium, which are essential for good cardiovascular health. Chuck bell peppers into salads or stir-fries to get lots of vitamin C and a good punch of antioxidants, or eat them as a snack between meals. Berries can be taken as the last course, which may combine blueberries, raspberries, and strawberries high in antioxidants and fiber, or they can be added to oatmeal or yogurt parfaits.

Lower sodium intake: The cardiologists recommend reducing sodium intake by removing the intake of processed and prepackaged foods and increasing the intake of a minimum amount of salt used in cooking and at the table. High levels of dietary sodium are a key contributing factor to high blood pressure, a significant risk factor for heart disease. Processed and pre-packaged food items—canned soups, frozen dinners, and snacks—are often loaded with extra sodium to preserve the food or to enhance its flavor. Look at the nutrition labels to find out your best options for low-sodium or sodium-free alternatives. Use herbs, spices, and lemon juice in your food for seasoning, not salt. With the great, intense flavor that such herbs as basil, cilantro, and parsley offer, you can use these without adding extra sodium. Cumin, paprika, and garlic powder can also give your food an extra taste without much-added salt.

Hydration: Nutritionists recommend a plentiful water supply to people during the day since dehydration could strain the cardiovascular system. It is essential for healthy blood volume and effective, efficient nutrient and oxygen transportation. Replace sugared drinks with unsweetened tea or sparkling water with fresh fruit slices. Be sure to bring your water bottle along. Drink water throughout the day and not when you reach the point where high-sugar, high-calorie beverages look too tempting to resist. If you do not like plain water, try it with some slices of fresh fruits, such as lemon, lime, or cucumber, which provides some flavor and keeps it refreshing without added calories or sugar.

Use healthy cooking methods: Cardiologists advocate for foods preferably baked, grilled, steamed, or sautéed with healthy oils like olive or avocado rather than deep-fried or foods prepared with high-calorie, unhealthy fats. Such is the skill in getting healthful flavor out of the meal without the pitfalls of saturated fats and calories from deep-frying or the addition of unhealthful fats. Wholesome and delicious possibilities would be to bake or grill lean proteins such as chicken, fish, or tofu. Sauté vegetables or proteins in minimal olive or avocado oil are good sources of monounsaturated fats. Steaming allows vegetables to be prepared gently, maintaining and preserving their nutrients and flavor. You can also experiment with tasty herbs and spices for flavor without additional fats or sodium. A heart-healthy diet should be individualized to what each person likes and needs; professional help is strongly encouraged to construct a plan that best fits into health goals and eating needs.

Be active: Many nutritionists and cardiologists would firmly state that apart from proper nutrition for the heart, the returns in maintaining sustained physical activity are very high. Routine physical activities, when done regularly, are highly effective in controlling and maintaining a healthy body weight, controlling the levels of blood pressure, and generally improving health status in the cardiovascular system. Moderate to vigorous physical activity, which includes aerobic exercises such as brisk walking, running, cycling, or swimming, is a very effective means of bringing blood pressure to the desired levels among people with hypertension. The heart can, therefore, pump at a reduced pressure for exercise compared to when it is at rest, which reduces the force that the blood has in the flow through the arteries and, in effect, the blood pressure. The regularity of physical activity results in the dependency of elasticity of the blood vessel, therefore significantly maintaining the improved blood pressure. Thus, exercise becomes all-important, resulting in great cardiovascular well-being and function. Regular physical activity keeps the heart muscle strong, allowing it to pump blood with less effort. It will be a bonus if the improved circulation reduces the risks of clotting or other cardiovascular issues. It also helps improve cholesterol levels by increasing HDL cholesterol while lowering LDL cholesterol. This beneficial effect on cholesterol levels reduces the possibility of plaque sticking to arteries and, as a result, decreases the chances of heart disease. Researchers have also discovered that exercise drastically lowers the body's inflammation levels, a significant cause of most chronic diseases, such as heart disease. Chronic inflammation inflicts an injury to the blood vessels, providing the base for plaque to build up and significantly increasing the risk of heart attacks and stroke. Hence, exercise minimizes inflammation and plays a vital role in cardiovascular health. Cardiologists and nutritionists emphasize that the importance of regular physical activity goes far beyond weight and blood pressure control. Exercise is associated with increased insulin sensitivity, a critical mechanism in blood-sugar regulation, and hence decreases the risk of contracting type 2 diabetes, a significant factor in heart diseases. It also reduces stress and improves heart health, as chronic stress predisposes individuals to high blood pressure, inflammation, and other heart problems.

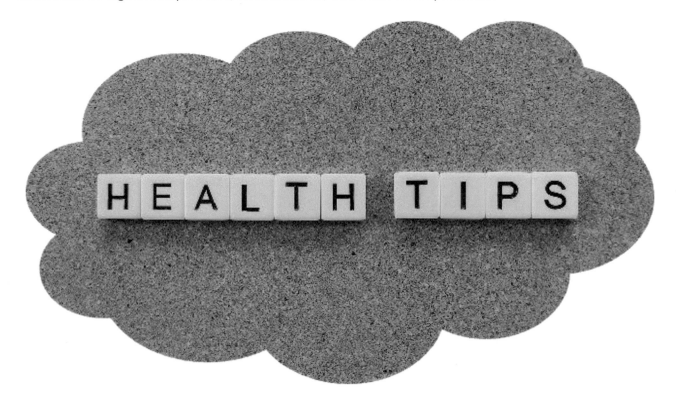

8.2 STAYING MOTIVATED ON YOUR DIET

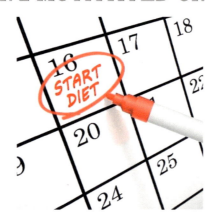

The most challenging part of any diet is not adopting it but staying motivated on your diet. Indeed, a study of people adopting a heart-healthy diet, published in 2019 in the Journal of Nutrition Education and Behavior, conducted interviews with 26 individuals diagnosed with cardiovascular disease or at high risk of cardiovascular disease. A person in this sample was 62-year-old Robert, who described how he kept himself motivated for the diet after having an MI. Robert related that at the outset, his motivation was to live longer for his family. It was helpful to have his wife with him on the journey to a diet for a healthy heart. They prepared meal plans, shopped in the market, and cooked at home to have nutritious meals. His wife was his accountability partner who inspired him at every impulse to consume something junk and recognized his success days with cheer and applause. Other factors that helped Robert stay motivated are the small yet measurable goals he defined for himself. He started by systematically removing junk from his diet, replacing some with fruits and vegetables. There was a sense of achievement that came with each goal, which drove him further to achieve more and make more positive changes in his life.

He also firmly pointed out that it has to be enjoyed throughout the process. He and his wife tried every method of preparing recipe after recipe, experimenting with tasty, satisfying ways to cook a heart-healthy diet. This food enjoyment made it easier for Robert to adhere to his dietary changes. Despite many temptations, Robert did not waver but stuck to the heart-healthy diet, which later benefitted him. He rewarded himself with non-food rewards, such as a weekend trip or a new book, to strengthen positive behaviors. Robert's work on a heart-healthy diet began to pay off: he started losing pounds, his cholesterol went down, and he started feeling way better. Here are a few ways to stay motivated and on your healthy diet plan:

Set realistic goals for yourself, such as gradually increasing your intake of fruits and vegetables or reducing your consumption of processed foods. Celebrate small victories along the way to keep yourself motivated.

Find an accountability partner: Have someone be there with you, a friend, family member, or support group with similar dietary goals. It keeps you in line and motivated. You might also find that you support and motivate each other, share healthy recipes, and celebrate your successes.

Make it enjoyable: Don't view your heart-healthy diet as a restrictive or punishing experience. Experiment with new recipes, cook in different ways and taste different flavors and cuisines that will make you healthy enough to achieve your dietary goal. Healthy eating can be delectable and very satisfying.

Meal prepping will help you keep your diet on track. Prior preparation is critical. This means setting aside time in the week to plan your meals, make a grocery list, and pre-cook some healthy snacks or meals so you don't have to start cooking at the last minute and ditch all your good intentions. This can avoid those late unhealthy options when you are out of time and starving.

Focus on benefits: Remind yourself of the many benefits a heart-healthy diet offers, such as improved energy, better sleep, and a lower risk of heart disease and stroke, among many other chronic diseases. Visualize how those benefits will add meaning to your life.

Treat yourself, but in moderation: Living with control, yet splurging sometimes helps take the edge off deprivation and makes the diet a sustained effort. Plan accordingly, with these indulgences in moderation, and then savor them mindfully.

Keep a food journal: Write everything down to help you be accountable and observe potential places to improve your eating. Use a food journal or an app to record what you eat and drink and review them regularly to become increasingly aware of your eating patterns and whether any changes need to be made.

Celebrate with non-food rewards: Instead of allowing food to be a reward, use non-food rewards—such as a massage or a new book—to learn the correct way to use food and to reinforce healthy behaviors.

Be Patient and Persistent. Changing dietary habits takes time and effort; therefore, be patient. Realize that there may be pitfalls or temporary lapses. With persistence, each good step you take is one step further in the right direction.

Note: Remember, achieving consistent motivation for a heart-healthy diet is a process. It is important to identify the most effective ways to do so. Support from health professionals, registered dietitians, or support groups can also help guide and encourage you.

8.3 ADJUSTING RECIPES FOR HEALTH

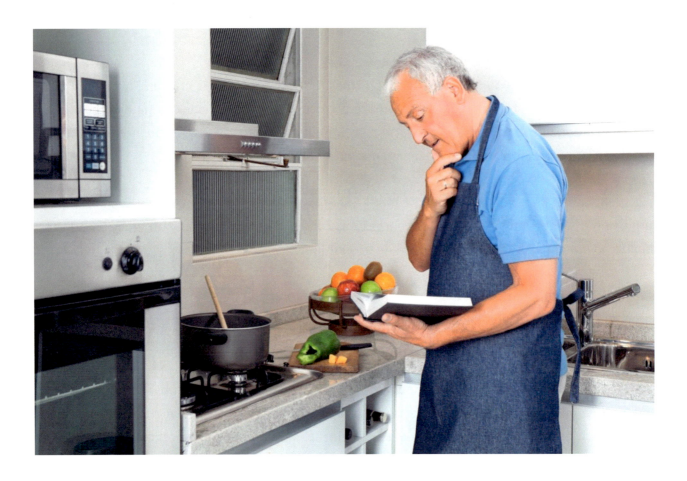

Meaningful modification of recipes flavor within a heart-healthy diet is a preventive measure. Indeed, adjusting Recipes for Health and Flavor that are thoughtfully made can help improve the nutritional quality of dishes, and can also help reduce harmful components and regulate body weight, and prevent the onset of chronic diseases while at the same time enhancing the general enjoyment of the foods. These changes do far more than improve the heart's health; they help ensure a fuller, more energetic life. Yet, we should never forget that a heart-healthy diet is not about deprivation but transformation; in that process, the experience of every daily meal should become joyful and filled with delight. So, making your favorite heart-healthy recipes doesn't have to mean sacrificing flavor. Here are some tips on how to adjust recipes for both health and deliciousness:

Fat Swaps: Reduce Overall Fat: Many recipes call for more fat than necessary. You can often reduce the amount of oil or butter by a third without affecting the taste or texture. For example, if a recipe calls for 1/2 cup of butter, try using 1/3 cup instead.

Choose Healthy Fats: Swap unhealthy saturated and trans fats for heart-healthy options. Replace butter with olive oil or avocado oil for cooking. Use lean protein sources like skinless chicken breast or fish instead of fatty meats.

Reduce Sodium: Salty sauces and processed ingredients can significantly increase sodium content. Look for low-sodium alternatives for broths, canned goods, and condiments.

Spice Up Your recipes: Instead of relying on salt for flavor, explore the vast world of herbs and spices. Experiment with different combinations to add complexity and depth to your dishes. Garlic, onion, chili powder, smoked paprika, and fresh herbs like rosemary and thyme are all fantastic options.
Acid is Your Friend: A squeeze of lemon juice or a splash of vinegar can brighten flavors and add a tangy touch, reducing your need for salt.

Whole Grains for the Win: Replace refined flours with whole-wheat flour or other whole grains in baked goods, pastas, and breading. Whole grains add fiber, which keeps you feeling full and promotes heart health. Start by substituting half the refined flour with a whole-grain option and gradually increase the whole-grain content as you get used to the texture.

Sugar Reduction: Satisfy your sweet tooth without overloading on sugar. Reduce the amount of sugar called for in recipes by 1/3 to 1/2. You might be surprised how little you actually need for a satisfying sweetness.
Natural Sweeteners: Experiment with natural sweeteners like pureed fruits (applesauce in muffins!), dates, or maple syrup for a healthier twist.

Note:
Remember to start small: Don't try to overhaul every recipe at once. Begin by making small adjustments and see how they affect the taste and texture. Gradually, you'll build your confidence and create heart-healthy versions of your favorite dishes. And don't forget to taste as you go: Don't be afraid to adjust seasonings as you cook. Adding a little more spice or a squeeze of lemon juice can make all the difference in achieving a flavorful and healthy dish.

By using these tips, you can transform your favorite recipes into heart-healthy meals that are both delicious and good for you.

CHAPTER 9: THE 30-DAY HEALTHY MEAL PLAN

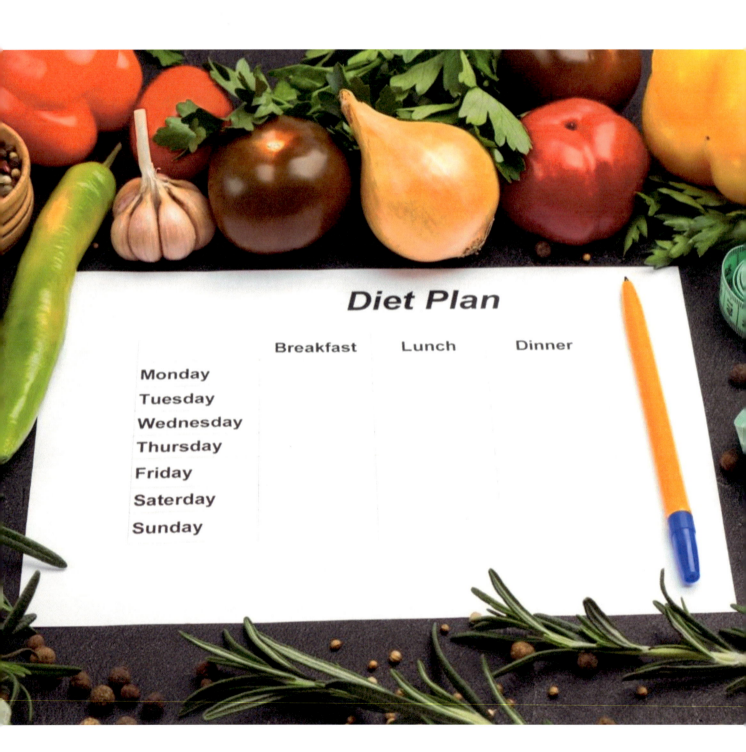

30-DAY HEART HEALTHY DIET MEAL PLAN

Day	Breakfast	Starter	Lunch	Snack	Dinner	Dessert
Day 1	Cinnamon Pancakes	Cucumber Bites	Classic Caesar Salad	Edamame with Twist	Baked Salmon with Lemon Dill Sauce	Oatmeal Cookies
Day 2	Breakfast Strata	Deviled Eggs	Southwestern Black Bean Salad	Roasted Chickpeas with Herbs	Herb-Crusted Chicken Breast	Chocolate-Fudge Pudding Cake
Day 3	Almond Chia Pudding	Bacon-Wrapped Avocado Fries	Kale and Blueberry Salad	Roasted Radishes	Veggie Tacos	Healthy Cookies
Day 4	Coconut Flour Waffles	Antipasto Skewers	Mediterranean Salad	Lentil Patties	Baked Cod	Meringues
Day 5	Salmon Scramble	Zucchini Roll-Ups with Goat Cheese	Citrus Avocado Salad with Pomegranate	Quinoa And Veggie Stuffed Mushrooms	Herb-Roasted Sweet Potatoes with Chicken	Apple Crisp
Day 6	Cauliflower Hash Browns	Avocado Boats with Tuna Salad	Anti-Oxidant Cabbage Salad	Baked Eggplant Fries	Baked Pesto Turkey Meatballs	Cinnamon-Raisin Oatmeal Cookies
Day 7	Coconut Yogurt Parfait	Sweet Potato Hash	Cauliflower Tabbouleh	Baked Pears with Walnuts	Chicken Breasts with Mango and Pineapple	Baked Apple Chips
Day 8	Smoked Salmon Frittata	Spicy Roasted Cauliflower	Avocado Spinach Salad	Roasted Butternut Squash	Chickpea and Cauliflower Curry	Strawberry-Banana Ice Cream
Day 9	Shakshuka	Spring Rolls	Zucchini Noodles Salad	Baked Zucchini Patties	Grilled Spicy Chicken Skewers	Grilled Peaches with Cinnamon Coconut Cream
Day 10	Mascarpone & Berries Toast	Stuffed Grape Leaves	Egg and Spinach Salad	Stuffed Figs Pockets	Poached Flounder with Ginger	Chocolate-Dipped Strawberry Bites
Day 11	Spinach and Chia Smoothie	Cucumber Bites	Butternut Squash Soup	Oatmeal Almond Bars	Stuffed Eggplant	Mint and Lime Fruit Salad
Day 12	Berry Smoothie	Deviled Eggs	Lentil Vegetable Soup	Pumpkin Bars	Lentil and Vegetable Loaf	Fruit Kabobs
Day 13	Peanut Butter	Bacon-Wrapped	Tomato Basil	Blueberry	Grilled Spicy Tuna	Spiced Baked

	Smoothie	Avocado Fries	Soup	Almond Bars	Steaks	Plums
Day 14	Coconut Smoothie	Antipasto Skewers	Chicken and Sweet Potato Soup	Oatmeal Almond Vanilla Bars	Vegetable and Tofu Kebabs with Peanut Sauce	Plum and Almond Tart
Day 15	Cocoa Avocado Smoothie	Zucchini Roll-Ups with Goat Cheese	Split Pea Soup	Chocolate Healthy Bars	Heart-Healthy Freekeh with Roasted Eggplant	Frozen Banana Pops
Day 16	Matcha Smoothie	Avocado Boats with Tuna Salad	Roasted Red Pepper and Tomato Soup	Carrot Healthy Bars	Spinach Falafel	Grapefruit Brûlée
Day 17	Vanilla Smoothie	Sweet Potato Hash	Mushroom and Barley Soup	Cranberry Orange Bars	Whole Wheat Pizza with Vegetables	Oatmeal Cookies
Day 18	Strawberry Smoothie	Spicy Roasted Cauliflower	Curried Cauliflower and Lentil Soup	Rolled Oats Flaxseed Bars	Cauliflower Wellington	Chocolate-Fudge Pudding Cake
Day 19	Coffee Smoothie	Spring Rolls	White Bean and Kale Soup with Rosemary	Blueberry Bars	Cauliflower Gnocchi	Healthy Cookies
Day 20	Raspberry Lemon Smoothie	Stuffed Grape Leaves	Tuscan-Style Vegetable and Chickpea Soup	Lemon Blueberry Cheesecake Bars	Mediterranean Grilled Vegetable Skewers	Meringues
Day 21	Cinnamon Pancakes	Cucumber Bites	Classic Caesar Salad	Oatmeal Almond Bars	Baked Salmon with Lemon Dill Sauce	Apple Crisp
Day 22	Breakfast Strata	Deviled Eggs	Southwestern Black Bean Salad	Roasted Chickpeas with Herbs	Herb-Crusted Chicken Breast	Cinnamon-Raisin Oatmeal Cookies
Day 23	Almond Chia Pudding	Bacon-Wrapped Avocado Fries	Kale and Blueberry Salad	Roasted Radishes	Veggie Tacos	Baked Apple Chips
Day 24	Coconut Flour Waffles	Antipasto Skewers	Mediterranean Salad	Lentil Patties	Baked Cod	Strawberry-Banana Ice Cream
Day 25	Salmon Scramble	Zucchini Roll-Ups with Goat Cheese	Citrus Avocado Salad with Pomegranate	Quinoa And Veggie Stuffed Mushrooms	Herb-Roasted Sweet Potatoes with Chicken	Grilled Peaches with Cinnamon Coconut Cream
Day 26	Cauliflower Hash Browns	Avocado Boats with Tuna Salad	Anti-Oxidant Cabbage Salad	Baked Eggplant Fries	Baked Pesto Turkey Meatballs	Chocolate-Dipped

136

					Strawberry Bites
Day 27	Coconut Yogurt Parfait	Sweet Potato Hash	Cauliflower Tabbouleh	Baked Pears with Walnuts	Chicken Breasts with Mango and Pineapple	Mint and Lime Fruit Salad
Day 28	Smoked Salmon Frittata	Spicy Roasted Cauliflower	Avocado Spinach Salad	Roasted Butternut Squash	Chickpea and Cauliflower Curry	Fruit Kabobs
Day 29	Shakshuka	Spring Rolls	Zucchini Noodles Salad	Baked Zucchini Patties	Grilled Spicy Chicken Skewers	Spiced Baked Plums
Day 30	Mascarpone & Berries Toast	Stuffed Grape Leaves	Egg and Spinach Salad	Stuffed Figs Pockets	Poached Flounder with Ginger	Plum and Al

30-DAY KETOGENIC DIET MEAL PLAN

Day	Breakfast	Starter	Lunch	Snack	Dinner	Dessert
Day 1	Avocado and egg bowl with spinach	Cucumber slices with guacamole	Grilled salmon salad with mixed greens, olive oil, and lemon dressing	Celery sticks with almond butter	Baked chicken thighs with roasted Brussels sprouts	Chia seed pudding with unsweetened almond milk and berries
Day 2	Greek yogurt with chia seeds and a handful of walnuts	Cherry tomatoes with mozzarella balls and basil	Turkey lettuce wraps with avocado and bell peppers	Olives and a small piece of dark chocolate (70% cocoa)	Zucchini noodles with pesto and grilled shrimp	Coconut flakes with a few raspberries
Day 3	Smoothie with spinach, avocado, unsweetened almond milk, and a scoop of protein powder	Bell pepper strips with hummus	Spinach and mushroom omelette with a side salad	Handful of macadamia nuts	Pork tenderloin with cauliflower mash	Lemon fat bombs (coconut oil, lemon zest, stevia)
Day 4	Scrambled eggs with smoked salmon and dill	Radishes with tzatziki	Chicken Caesar salad with homemade dressing (Greek yogurt base)	Small avocado with sea salt	Beef stir-fry with broccoli and bell peppers	Keto chocolate mug cake (almond flour, cocoa powder, stevia)
Day 5	Almond flour pancakes with a dollop of Greek yogurt and berries	Broccoli florets with cheese dip	Tuna salad with avocado and mixed greens	Hard-boiled eggs	Grilled lamb chops with asparagus	Strawberries with whipped coconut cream
Day 6	Cottage cheese with sliced almonds and a few blackberries	Sliced cucumber with cottage cheese dip	Egg salad lettuce wraps	A handful of pecans	Baked cod with lemon and garlic, served with a side of green beans	Keto coconut macaroons
Day 7	Keto smoothie bowl with spinach, avocado, and coconut milk	Cherry tomatoes with feta cheese	Grilled chicken and avocado salad with olive oil dressing	Pumpkin seeds	Turkey meatballs with zoodles (zucchini noodles)	Dark chocolate squares
Day 8	Bacon and egg breakfast muffins	Green bell pepper slices with cream cheese	Shrimp and avocado salad	Sliced deli meat with a cheese stick	Baked salmon with a side of spinach	Keto cheesecake bites
Day 9	Greek yogurt with chia seeds and a handful of walnuts	Cucumber slices with guacamole	Turkey lettuce wraps with avocado and bell peppers	Olives and a small piece of dark chocolate (70% cocoa)	Zucchini noodles with pesto and grilled shrimp	Coconut flakes with a few raspberries
Day 10	Scrambled eggs with smoked salmon and dill	Radishes with tzatziki	Chicken Caesar salad with homemade dressing (Greek yogurt base)	Small avocado with sea salt	Beef stir-fry with broccoli and bell peppers	Keto chocolate mug cake (almond flour, cocoa powder, stevia)
Day 11	Almond flour pancakes with a dollop of Greek yogurt and berries	Broccoli florets with cheese dip	Tuna salad with avocado and mixed greens	Hard-boiled eggs	Grilled lamb chops with asparagus	Strawberries with whipped coconut cream
Day 12	Cottage cheese with sliced almonds and a few blackberries	Sliced cucumber with cottage cheese dip	Egg salad lettuce wraps	A handful of pecans	Baked cod with lemon and garlic, served with a side of green beans	Keto coconut macaroons
Day	Keto smoothie bowl	Cherry	Grilled chicken	Pumpkin seeds	Turkey meatballs	Dark chocolate

13	with spinach, avocado, and coconut milk	tomatoes with feta cheese	and avocado salad with olive oil dressing		with zoodles (zucchini noodles)	squares
Day 14	Bacon and egg breakfast muffins	Green bell pepper slices with cream cheese	Shrimp and avocado salad	Sliced deli meat with a cheese stick	Baked salmon with a side of spinach	Keto cheesecake bites
Day 15	Avocado and egg bowl with spinach	Cucumber slices with guacamole	Grilled salmon salad with mixed greens, olive oil, and lemon dressing	Celery sticks with almond butter	Baked chicken thighs with roasted Brussels sprouts	Chia seed pudding with unsweetened almond milk and berries
Day 16	Greek yogurt with chia seeds and a handful of walnuts	Cherry tomatoes with mozzarella balls and basil	Turkey lettuce wraps with avocado and bell peppers	Olives and a small piece of dark chocolate (70% cocoa)	Zucchini noodles with pesto and grilled shrimp	Coconut flakes with a few raspberries
Day 17	Smoothie with spinach, avocado, unsweetened almond milk, and a scoop of protein powder	Bell pepper strips with hummus	Spinach and mushroom omelette with a side salad	Handful of macadamia nuts	Pork tenderloin with cauliflower mash	Lemon fat bombs (coconut oil, lemon zest, stevia)
Day 18	Scrambled eggs with smoked salmon and dill	Radishes with tzatziki	Chicken Caesar salad with homemade dressing (Greek yogurt base)	Small avocado with sea salt	Beef stir-fry with broccoli and bell peppers	Keto chocolate mug cake (almond flour, cocoa powder, stevia)
Day 19	Almond flour pancakes with a dollop of Greek yogurt and berries	Broccoli florets with cheese dip	Tuna salad with avocado and mixed greens	Hard-boiled eggs	Grilled lamb chops with asparagus	Strawberries with whipped coconut cream
Day 20	Cottage cheese with sliced almonds and a few blackberries	Sliced cucumber with cottage cheese dip	Egg salad lettuce wraps	A handful of pecans	Baked cod with lemon and garlic, served with a side of green beans	Keto coconut macaroons
Day 21	Keto smoothie bowl with spinach, avocado, and coconut milk	Cherry tomatoes with feta cheese	Grilled chicken and avocado salad with olive oil dressing	Pumpkin seeds	Turkey meatballs with zoodles (zucchini noodles)	Dark chocolate squares
Day 22	Bacon and egg breakfast muffins	Green bell pepper slices with cream cheese	Shrimp and avocado salad	Sliced deli meat with a cheese stick	Baked salmon with a side of spinach	Keto cheesecake bites
Day 23	Greek yogurt with chia seeds and a handful of walnuts	Cucumber slices with guacamole	Turkey lettuce wraps with avocado and bell peppers	Olives and a small piece of dark chocolate (70% cocoa)	Zucchini noodles with pesto and grilled shrimp	Coconut flakes with a few raspberries
Day 24	Scrambled eggs with smoked salmon and dill	Radishes with tzatziki	Chicken Caesar salad with homemade dressing (Greek yogurt base)	Small avocado with sea salt	Beef stir-fry with broccoli and bell peppers	Keto chocolate mug cake (almond flour, cocoa powder, stevia)
Day 25	Almond flour pancakes with a dollop of Greek yogurt and berries	Broccoli florets with cheese dip	Tuna salad with avocado and mixed greens	Hard-boiled eggs	Grilled lamb chops with asparagus	Strawberries with whipped coconut cream
Day 26	Cottage cheese with sliced almonds and a few blackberries	Sliced cucumber with cottage cheese	Egg salad lettuce wraps	A handful of pecans	Baked cod with lemon and garlic, served with a	Keto coconut macaroons

			dip			side of green beans	
Day 27	Keto smoothie bowl with spinach, avocado, and coconut milk	Cherry tomatoes with feta cheese	Grilled chicken and avocado salad with olive oil dressing	Pumpkin seeds	Turkey meatballs with zoodles (zucchini noodles)	Dark chocolate squares
Day 28	Bacon and egg breakfast muffins	Green bell pepper slices with cream cheese	Shrimp and avocado salad	Sliced deli meat with a cheese stick	Baked salmon with a side of spinach	Keto cheesecake bites
Day 29	Avocado and egg bowl with spinach	Cucumber slices with guacamole	Grilled salmon salad with mixed greens, olive oil, and lemon dressing	Celery sticks with almond butter	Baked chicken thighs with roasted Brussels sprouts	Chia seed pudding with unsweetened almond milk and berries
Day 30	Greek yogurt with chia seeds and a handful of walnuts	Cherry tomatoes with mozzarella balls and basil	Turkey lettuce wraps with avocado and bell peppers	Olives and a small piece of dark chocolate (70% cocoa)	Zucchini noodles with pesto and grilled shrimp	Coconut flakes with a few raspberries

140

30-DAY VEGETARIAN MEAL PLAN

Day	Breakfast	Starter	Lunch	Snack	Dinner	Dessert
Day 1	Avocado Toast with Cherry Tomatoes	Greek Yogurt with Honey and Nuts	Quinoa Salad with Black Beans and Corn	Carrot Sticks with Hummus	Grilled Portobello Mushrooms with Pesto	Fresh Fruit Salad
Day 2	Smoothie Bowl with Berries and Granola	Caprese Skewers	Lentil Soup with Spinach	Apple Slices with Almond Butter	Stuffed Bell Peppers with Quinoa	Dark Chocolate Squares
Day 3	Oatmeal with Banana and Chia Seeds	Cucumber Bites with Cream Cheese	Mediterranean Chickpea Salad	Mixed Nuts	Eggplant Parmesan	Baked Pears with Cinnamon
Day 4	Greek Yogurt Parfait with Berries	Spinach and Artichoke Dip with Whole Grain Crackers	Butternut Squash Soup	Edamame	Veggie Stir-Fry with Tofu	Chia Seed Pudding
Day 5	Smoothie with Kale, Pineapple, and Coconut Milk	Bruschetta with Tomato and Basil	Cauliflower Tacos with Avocado	Roasted Chickpeas	Spinach and Ricotta Stuffed Shells	Frozen Banana Bites
Day 6	Whole Grain Pancakes with Maple Syrup	Greek Salad	Sweet Potato and Black Bean Burrito Bowl	Bell Pepper Strips with Hummus	Vegetable Curry with Brown Rice	Coconut Macaroons
Day 7	Chia Pudding with Mango	Marinated Olives and Feta	Minestrone Soup	Popcorn with Nutritional Yeast	Grilled Vegetable Skewers	Raspberry Sorbet
Day 8	Avocado Smoothie	Tomato and Mozzarella Skewers	Kale Caesar Salad	Celery Sticks with Peanut Butter	Spaghetti Squash with Marinara Sauce	Fruit Yogurt
Day 9	Overnight Oats with Blueberries	Zucchini Fritters	Chickpea and Avocado Sandwich	Trail Mix	Vegetable Paella	Lemon Sorbet
Day 10	Scrambled Tofu with Spinach	Roasted Garlic and Herb Cashew Cheese	Tomato Basil Soup	Sunflower Seeds	Stuffed Zucchini Boats	Strawberry Shortcake
Day 11	Smoothie with Spinach, Mango, and Coconut Water	Caprese Salad	Roasted Beet and Goat Cheese Salad	Almonds	Thai Green Curry with Tofu	Coconut Milk Ice Cream
Day 12	Greek Yogurt with Mixed Berries	Carrot and Cucumber Sticks with Tzatziki	Vegetable Sushi Rolls	Roasted Edamame	Grilled Tofu Steaks	Chocolate Avocado Mousse
Day 13	Whole Grain Toast with Peanut Butter and Banana	Spinach and Feta Stuffed Mushrooms	Broccoli Cheddar Soup	Veggie Chips	Ratatouille	Peach Cobbler
Day 14	Oatmeal with Almond Butter and Berries	Kale Chips	Avocado and Quinoa Salad	Roasted Almonds	Eggplant Lasagna	Cherry Almond Cake
Day 15	Smoothie with Berries and Spinach	Cucumber and Tomato Salad	Lentil Stew	Pistachios	Stuffed Bell Peppers	Apple Crisp
Day 16	Chia Seed Pudding with Raspberries	Greek Yogurt with Honey and Walnuts	Chickpea Salad Wrap	Baby Carrots with Hummus	Roasted Vegetable Pizza	Pineapple Sorbet

141

Day 17	Avocado Toast with Red Pepper Flakes	Garlic Parmesan Roasted Cauliflower	Tomato Basil Quinoa	Mixed Fruit	Spinach and Mushroom Risotto	Chocolate Dipped Strawberries
Day 18	Smoothie Bowl with Banana and Granola	Stuffed Grape Leaves	Vegetable Pho	Cashews	Veggie Fajitas	Mango Sorbet
Day 19	Whole Grain Waffles with Berries	Greek Salad	Lentil and Sweet Potato Curry	Kale Chips	Zucchini Noodles with Pesto	Chia Pudding with Passionfruit
Day 20	Greek Yogurt with Granola and Honey	Roasted Red Pepper Hummus with Veggies	Black Bean Soup	Seaweed Snacks	Baked Eggplant Parmesan	Fresh Berry Compote
Day 21	Smoothie with Avocado and Pineapple	Tomato and Mozzarella Bruschetta	Roasted Vegetable Salad	Pumpkin Seeds	Stuffed Acorn Squash	Apple Cinnamon Muffins
Day 22	Chia Pudding with Blueberries	Greek Yogurt with Pomegranate	Spinach and Feta Quesadilla	Grapes and Cheese	Tofu and Vegetable Stir-Fry	Vegan Chocolate Cake
Day 23	Avocado and Tomato Toast	Hummus and Veggie Platter	Butternut Squash and Quinoa Salad	Spicy Roasted Chickpeas	Vegetable Moussaka	Mixed Berry Crumble
Day 24	Smoothie with Spinach, Apple, and Ginger	Caprese Salad	Lentil and Vegetable Stew	Almond Butter with Apple Slices	Stuffed Portobello Mushrooms	Coconut Rice Pudding
Day 25	Greek Yogurt with Almonds and Honey	Carrot and Cucumber Sticks with Hummus	Roasted Beet Salad	Trail Mix	Vegetable Tikka Masala	Lemon Bars
Day 26	Oatmeal with Fresh Berries	Bruschetta with Tomato and Basil	Chickpea and Spinach Salad	Cashews	Eggplant Rollatini	Chocolate Covered Bananas
Day 27	Smoothie with Blueberries and Almond Milk	Greek Yogurt with Nuts and Honey	Quinoa and Black Bean Salad	Bell Pepper Strips with Hummus	Grilled Vegetable Platter	Raspberry Sorbet
Day 28	Avocado Toast with Lemon and Salt	Stuffed Mushrooms	Lentil Soup with Kale	Almonds	Veggie Stir-Fry with Cashews	Coconut Macaroons
Day 29	Greek Yogurt with Fresh Fruit	Caprese Skewers	Roasted Sweet Potato and Black Bean Tacos	Roasted Chickpeas	Spinach and Ricotta Stuffed Shells	Frozen Grapes
Day 30	Smoothie Bowl with Spinach and Berries	Spinach and Artichoke Dip with Whole Grain Crackers	Tomato Basil Soup	Edamame	Veggie Lasagna	Fresh Fruit Salad

142

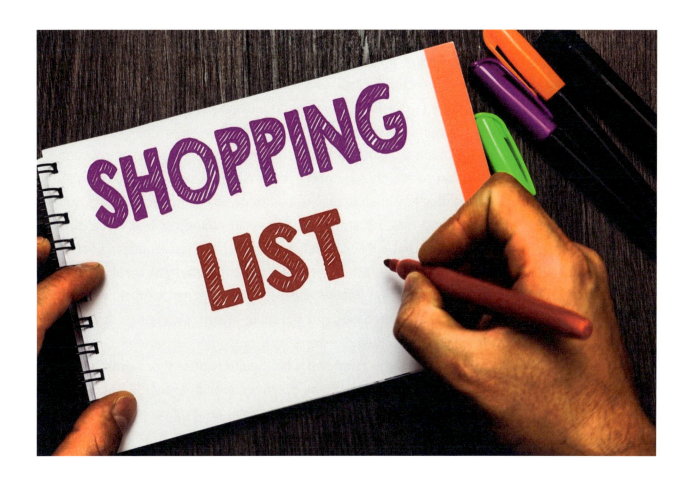

Weekly shopping lists and meal prepping are two powerful ways to stick to a heart-healthy diet. It has also always been a consistent con that many people adhere to nutritional guidelines and do better in cardiovascular health because they plan what to eat and cook at home. A study published in the American Journal of Preventive Medicine 2018 showed increased consumption of salads, fruit, and vegetables among individuals spending time on home food preparation. Also, this research identified that individuals spending less than one hour per day on food preparation reported high intake of fast foods and were more likely to use out-of-home food sources, increasing calorie consumption and having an overall poor nutrient profile. This means that the benefits of meal planning are far-reaching. These facts were explicitly put across by a systematic review in the International Journal of Behavioral Nutrition and Physical Activity, which reiterated that meal planning was associated with a healthier diet and lower body mass index—both crucial parts of heart health. According to this review, meal planners had a more balanced variety of food and showed a decreased likelihood of being overweight or obese. This is because obesity is said to be one of the high-risk factors when it comes to cardiovascular diseases; hence, meal planning and portion control can lead to the maintenance of a healthy weight, in which case such health issues are highly reduced. More important, however, is that sodium intake heavily determines one's heart health, and people can effectively manage their salt intake by eating home-cooked foods. The Centers for Disease Control and Prevention reports that more than 70% of sodium in the American diet comes from processed and restaurant foods. Making a detailed grocery list of whole, unprocessed ingredients and preparing those at home into meals can help minimize that added consumption. A study in the Journal of the Academy of Nutrition and Dietetics found that people who prepared meals at home six to seven times a week consumed about 137 fewer calories per day and 3 grams less fat than those who cooked dinner once a week or less. This reduction in calorie and fat uptake can eventually lead to massive improvements in the lipid profiles of patients, along with lowering high blood pressure levels over time. The psychological benefits of meal planning are also favorable for heart health. Chronic stress has been known to put patients at higher risk for hypertension, atherosclerosis, and overall cardiovascular diseases. An American Psychological Association survey found that 27% of adults miss meals due to stress, while 33% overeat or eat unhealthily. Through planning and preparation, an individual can be relieved from the countless daily decisions on what to eat, thus reducing stress and making other food choices with mindfulness. This mindfulness in eating has been associated with low BMI and good dietary quality in many research papers. Fiscally related matters are also at stake in dining for heart health. A U.S. Department of Agriculture study stated that approximately half of the average American's food dollar is spent on food eaten away from home. Regrettably, more frequent restaurant meal consumption positively relates to average total daily energy intake and negatively relates to diet quality. More specifically, investing the time to plan out purchases and shopping lists according to a concrete meal plan is way more economical. This affordability enables the customer to purchase quality and nourishing ingredients to contribute towards cardiovascular health without compromising family budgets. Besides, the dynamics associated with meal planning within a family should not be underestimated. According to the Journal of Nutrition Education and Behavior Research, kids participating in cooking lessons are more likely to crave fruits and vegetables. By preparing shopping lists and meals every week, money and time will not be wasted, and in the entire family, people will have developed healthy eating habits since childhood. A heart-healthy diet will not be complete without shopping lists and meal prepping every week. Associated practices can encompass better nutrient intake, improved management of weight, reduction in sodium consumption, less stress, mindfulness in eating, savings, and positively impacting family health behaviors. Meal planning, detailed shopping lists, and food preparation in advance are investments that any person makes in making active strides toward reducing the risks of cardiovascular disease and investing in long-term heart health.

9.1 HEART HEALTHY DIET SHOPPING LIST:

Week 1: Days 1-7

❖ **Proteins:**

- 6 fillets of salmon (for scramble, baked salmon, and rolls)
- 24 large eggs (for deviled eggs, strata, and scrambled eggs)
- 3 boneless chicken breasts
- 8 oz of low sodium. Bacon
- 2 (five oz.) cans of tuna
  ❖ **Dairy:**

- 1-pint Greek yogurt
- 1-quart almond milk
- 8 oz mascarpone cheese
- 8 oz goat cheese
- 8 ounces cream cheese
- 8 oz Parmesan cheese
- 16 ounces mozzarella cheese (for rolls)

❖ **Vegetables:**

- 4 avocados
- 4 large cucumbers
- 6 bell peppers
- 8 zucchinis
- 1 bunch radishes
- 2 heads cauliflower
- 2 large eggplants
- 2 bunches kale
- 2 bags of baby spinach

- 2 heads of romaine lettuce
- 1 pint of cherry tomatoes
- 1 butternut squash
- 8 oz mushrooms
- 4 portobello mushrooms
- 2 sweet potatoes
- 6 jalapeños

❖ **Fruits:**

- 6 lemons
- 1-pint strawberries
- 1-pint blueberries
- 4 peaches
- 6 apples
- 4 bananas

❖ **Pantry Items:**

- 1 lb quinoa
- 8 oz. Chia seeds
- 2 cups coconut flour
- 2 cups almond flour
- 1 quart olive oil
- 1 pint coconut oil
- 16 oz almond butter
- 16 ounces hummus
- 1 lb mixed nuts (almonds, walnuts)

❖ **Fresh herbs:**

- 1 bunch of dill, basil, and parsley
- Spices: 1 jar every of cinnamon, cumin, and paprika
- 1 quart apple cider vinegar
- 1-quart balsamic vinegar

❖ **Others:**

- 1 lb edamame
- nori sheets (optional)
- 1 loaf whole grain bread
- 1 box whole grain crackers

Week 2: Days 8-14

❖ **Proteins:**

- 12 large eggs
- 3 boneless chicken breasts
- 8 ounces bacon
- 6 fillets of salmon
- 16 oz lentils

❖ **Dairy:**

- 1 pint Greek yogurt
- 1-quart almond milk
- 8 oz cream cheese
- 8 ounces of Parmesan cheese

❖ **Vegetables:**

- 4 avocados
- 4 cucumbers
- 6 bell peppers
- 8 zucchinis
- 1 bunch radishes
- 2 heads cauliflower
- 2 large eggplants
- 2 bunches kale
- 2 bunches of spinach
- 2 heads of romaine lettuce

- 1 pint of cherry tomatoes
- 1 butternut squash
- 8 oz mushrooms
- 4 portobello mushrooms
- 2 candy potatoes
- 6 jalapeños

❖ **Fruits:**

- 6 lemons
- 1-pint strawberries
- 1-pint blueberries
- 4 peaches
- 6 apples
- 4 bananas

❖ **Pantry Items:**

- 8 oz chia seeds
- 2 cups coconut flour
- 2 cups almond flour
- 1 quart olive oil
- 1 pint coconut oil
- 16 oz Almond butter
- 16 oz hummus
- 1 lb combined nuts (almonds, walnuts)
- Fresh herbs: 1 bunch of dill, basil, and parsley
- Spices: 1 jar each of cinnamon, cumin, paprika
- 1 quart apple cider vinegar
- 1-quart balsamic vinegar

❖ **Others:**

- 1 lb edamame
- 1 percent nori sheets (non-obligatory)
- 1 loaf whole grain bread
- 1 container of complete grain crackers

Week 3: Days 15-21

❖ **Proteins:**

- 12 huge eggs
- three boneless hen breasts
- 8 ounces bacon
- 2 (5 oz) cans of tuna
- 6 fillets of salmon
- 16 oz lentils

❖ **Dairy:**

- 1 pint Greek yogurt
- 1-quart almond milk
- 8oz.Cream cheese
- 8oz cheese

❖ **Vegetables:**

- 4 avocados
- 4 large cucumbers
- 6 bell peppers
- 8 zucchinis
- 1 bunch radishes
- 2 heads cauliflower
- 2 large eggplants
- 2 bunches kale
- 2 bunches of baby spinach
- 2 heads of romaine lettuce
- 1 pint of cherry tomatoes
- 1 butternut squash
- 8 oz mushrooms
- 4portobello mushrooms
- 2 sweet potatoes
- 6 jalapeños

❖ **Fruits:**

- 6 lemons
- 1-pint strawberries
- 1-pint blueberries
- 4 peaches
- 6 apples
- 4 bananas

❖ **Pantry Items:**

- 8 oz chia seeds
- 2 cups coconut flour
- 2 cups almond flour
- 1 quart olive oil
- 1 pint coconut oil
- 16 oz. Almond butter
- 16 oz. Hummus
- 1 lb combined nuts (almonds, walnuts)
- Fresh herbs: 1 bunch of dill, basil, and parsley
- Spices: 1 jar of cinnamon, cumin, paprika
- 1 quart apple cider vinegar
- 1-quart balsamic vinegar

❖ **Others:**

- 1 lb edamame
- 1 loaf of complete grain bread
- whole grain crackers

Week 4: Days 22-30

❖ **Proteins:**

- 12 large eggs
- 3 boneless fowl breasts
- 8oz of Bacon
- 6 fillets of salmon
- 16 ounces lentils

❖ **Dairy:**

- 1-pint Greek yogurt
- 1-quart almond milk
- 8 ounces cream cheese
- 8oz.Parmesan cheese

❖ **Vegetables:**

- 4avocados
- 4 large cucumbers
- 6 bell peppers
- 8 zucchinis
- 1 bunch radishes
- 2 heads cauliflower
- 2 large eggplants
- 2 bunches kale
- 2 bunches of baby spinach
- 2 heads of romaine lettuce
- 1 pint of cherry tomatoes
- 1 butternut squash
- 8 oz mushrooms
- 4 portobello mushrooms
- 2 sweet potatoes

- 6 jalapeños

❖ **Fruits:**

- 6 lemons
- 1-pint strawberries
- 1-pint blueberries
- 4 peaches
- 6 apples
- 4 bananas

❖ **Pantry Items:**

- 8 oz of. Chia seeds
- 2 cups coconut flour
- 2 cups almond flour
- 1 quart olive oil
- 1 pint coconut oil
- 16 Oz. Almond butter
- 16 oz. Hummus

- 1 lb blended nuts (almonds, walnuts)
- Fresh herbs: 1 bunch each of dill, basil, and parsley
- Spices: 1 jar each of cinnamon, cumin, paprika
- 1 quart apple cider vinegar
- 1-quart balsamic vinegar

❖ **Others:**

- 1 lb edamame
- nori sheets (optionally available)
- 1 loaf whole grain bread
- 1 box of whole-grain crackers

CHAPTER 10: HEART-HEALTHY FOOD MIX IDEAS

For delicious and nutritious weeknight dinners, we can try the following heart-healthy food combinations that convey colorful flavors and provide beneficial vitamins for our bodies. Whether you are in the mood for seafood, poultry, vegetarian, or a combination of different protein sources, these innovative mixtures are designed to make your meals fun and beneficial for healthy heart fitness. Here are great food blend ideas and creative combinations to inspire your meal-making plans:

Combo #	Heart-Healthy Food Mix Ideas
1	Grilled Salmon with Lemon Dill Sauce + Quinoa and Black Bean Bowl
2	Chicken and Sweet Potato Soup + Kale and Blueberry Salad
3	Vegetable and Tofu Kebabs with Peanut Sauce + Cauliflower Tabbouleh
4	Baked Cod with Mediterranean Salsa + Herb-Roasted Sweet Potatoes
5	Spinach Falafel + Butternut Squash Soup
6	Pesto-Crusted Sea Bass + Zucchini Noodles Salad
7	Lentil and Vegetable Loaf + Garlic Roasted Green Beans
8	Grilled Spicy Tuna Steaks + Citrus Avocado Salad
9	Stuffed Eggplant + Whole Wheat Pizza with Vegetables
10	Herb-crusted chicken Breast + Barley and Lentil Loaf
11	Macadamia Nut Crusted Mahi Mahi + Avocado Spinach Salad
12	Steamed Halibut + Classic Caesar Salad
13	Baked Cod + Mediterranean Grilled Vegetable Skewers
14	Spicy Grilled Tuna Steaks + Anti-Oxidant Cabbage Salad
15	Stuffed Grape Leaves + White Bean and Kale Soup with Rosemary
16	Broiled Mackerel with Ginger and Green Onions + Quinoa and Veggie Stuffed Mushrooms
17	Grilled Spicy Chicken Skewers + Citrus Avocado Salad
18	Herb-crusted chicken Breast + Butternut Squash and Sage Barley Risotto
19	Chicken Breasts with Mango and Pineapple + Spinach and Avocado Salad
20	Turkey Veggie Lettuce Wraps + Lemon Herb Couscous
21	Lentil Walnut Veggie Burgers + Anti-Oxidant Cabbage Salad

22	Cauliflower Gnocchi + Zucchini Noodles Salad
23	Stuffed Sweet Potatoes + Tuscan-style vegetable and Chickpea Soup
24	Roasted Red Pepper and Tomato Soup + Spinach Falafel
25	Pesto-Crusted Sea Bass + Grilled Corn and Black Bean Salsa
26	Baked Pesto Turkey Meatballs + Split Pea Soup
27	Cauliflower Wellington + Southwestern Black Bean Salad
28	Spinach Falafel + Butternut Squash Soup
29	Veggie Tacos + Avocado Spinach Salad

10.1. CREATIVE COMBOS FOR WEEKNIGHT DINNERS

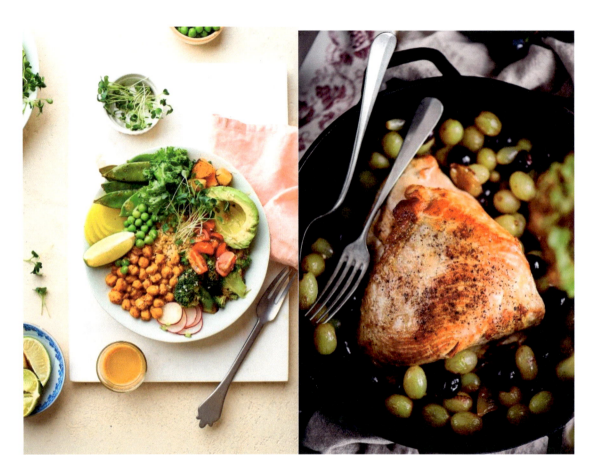

Creative weeknight dinner combos are a fantastic way to get out of a classic dinner dish and include some excitement into your everyday life without spending hours slaving over dinner. The trick: Re-envision familiar ingredients and merge different culinary traditions, making unique and satisfying meals. For instance, turning that sweet potato into a taco filling makes it exponentially more nutritious and ensures that Taco Tuesday is at least twice as fun. Creative fusions, such as Greek-style quesadillas or Asian lettuce wraps, blend delicious flavors and textures, which taste buds on a trip worldwide. "Breakfast for dinner" takes on new meaning and is the gateway to protein-packed frittatas and savory waffles at the end of the day. Adding simple cooking techniques such as one-pan skillet meals and foil-packet dinners can cut time for preparation and cleanup in half without sacrificing taste or nutrition. Think of adding plant-based alternatives like cauliflower rice or zucchini noodles, adding tons of extra volume and nutrients to your meal without weighing it down. The beauty is in their flexibility: many can be easily adapted to use leftover ingredients, comply with dietary preferences, or showcase seasonal produce. By thinking outside the box and combining unexpected elements, you can turn everyday ingredients into exciting, restaurant-worthy meals that will have your family looking forward to dinnertime all week long. Here are some of the most creative combos that you can enjoy during weeknight dinners

Combo #	Creative Combos for Weeknight Dinners
1	Zesty Baked Trout + Spinach and Avocado Salad
2	Stuffed Bell Peppers + Mushroom and Barley Risotto
3	Spicy Grilled Chicken Skewers + Cauliflower Gnocchi
4	Poached Flounder with Ginger + Couscous and Barley with Veggies
5	Baked Pesto Turkey Meatballs + Curried Cauliflower and Lentil Soup
6	Broiled Mackerel with Ginger and Green Onions + Millet and Roasted Vegetable Bowl
7	Chicken Masala + Anti-Oxidant Cabbage Salad
8	Veggie Tacos + Balsamic Glazed Roasted Root Vegetables
9	Cauliflower Wellington + Citrus Avocado Salad
10	Stuffed Sweet Potatoes + Tuscan-style vegetable and Chickpea Soup
11	Lemon Herb Couscous + Grilled Vegetable Skewers
12	Broiled Mackerel with Ginger and Green Onions + Zucchini Noodles Salad
13	Quinoa and Veggie Stuffed Mushrooms + Roasted Butternut Squash
14	Roasted Chickpeas with Herbs + Mushroom and Spinach Barley Risotto
15	Baked Eggplant Fries + Southwestern Black Bean Salad
16	Spinach Falafel + Lentil and Vegetable Loaf
17	Lentil Patties + Mediterranean Grilled Vegetable Skewers
18	Smashed Zucchini with Pesto & Burrata + Chicken and Sweet Potato Soup
19	Macadamia Nut Crusted Mahi + Avocado Mash
20	Baked Pears with Walnuts + Lemon Tahini Dressing
21	Herb Roasted Portabella Mushrooms + Citrus Avocado Salad
22	Steamed Halibut + Anti-Oxidant Cabbage Salad
23	Cauliflower Wellington + Curried Eggplants
24	Roasted Butternut Squash + Avocado Spinach Salad
25	Stuffed Bell Peppers + Kale and Blueberry Salad
26	Stuffed Eggplant + Cauliflower Tabbouleh
27	Chicken Masala + Citrus Avocado Salad
28	Vegetable and Tofu Kebabs with Peanut Sauce + Grilled Corn and Black Bean Salsa
29	Stuffed Sweet Potatoes + Butternut Squash Soup
30	Lentil and Vegetable Loaf + Garlic Roasted Green Beans

10.2. MIX AND MATCH MEAL PLANNING

Mix-and-match meal planning entails an innovative way of structuring meals with various ingredients that can be mixed and matched to create many healthy and satisfying dishes. In this way, you can easily prepare together your foods to create any diverse and exciting dishes you have in mind, avoiding boredom with your diet and poor nutrition. There are numerous vital elements of mix-and-match meal planning flexibility: You can select from various ingredients and combine them based on what you like, what you need for dietary reasons, and what is in your kitchen.

You can also create many meal variations, which would help avoid monotony in the diet and bring different nutrients to the plate.

Keeping your meals simple makes meal preparation and planning easy, thus allowing you to achieve proper time and resource management in maintaining a healthy diet.

There are various advantages of Mix and Match Meal Planning, including.

Personalization. Prepare meals according to your preferences, dietary limitations, and nutritional requirements.

Besides, it would be best to streamline grocery shopping and meal prep by focusing on versatile ingredients. By the end of the day, Match Meal Planning plays a vital role in promoting healthy eating; it encourages the consumption of various nutrient-dense foods.

And here are some of the best ways that can help us Mix and Match Meal Planning:

Breakfast Options

Option	Base	Toppings/Extras
Oatmeal Delight	1 cup of oatmeal	Fresh berries, a handful of nuts, a drizzle of honey
Greek Yogurt Parfait	1 cup non-fat Greek yogurt	Sliced bananas, sprinkle of granola, chia seeds
Veggie Omelette	2 egg whites	Spinach, tomatoes, mushrooms, onions
Whole Grain Toast	2 slices whole-grain toast	Avocado, sliced tomato, sprinkle of flax seeds
Smoothie Bowl	1 cup blended fruit	Fresh fruit slices, almonds, shredded coconut

Lunch Options

Option	Base	Toppings/Extras
Quinoa Salad	1 cup cooked quinoa	Chopped cucumbers, cherry tomatoes, feta cheese, olive oil
Turkey Wrap	Whole grain tortilla	Sliced turkey, lettuce, avocado, mustard
Lentil Soup	1 cup lentil soup	Spinach, diced carrots, celery, a dash of lemon juice
Mixed Green Salad	Mixed greens	Grilled chicken, walnuts, cranberries, balsamic vinaigrette
Brown Rice Bowl	1 cup brown rice	Black beans, corn, salsa, diced red peppers

Snack Options

Option	Base	Toppings/Extras
Apple Slices	Sliced apple	Almond butter, sprinkle of cinnamon
Carrot Sticks	Carrot sticks	Hummus
Nuts & Seeds Mix	Handful of mixed nuts	Dried cranberries, pumpkin seeds
Rice Cakes	Whole grain rice cakes	Peanut butter, banana slices
Cottage Cheese	1 cup cottage cheese	Pineapple chunks, sunflower seeds

Dinner Options

Option	Base	Toppings/Extras
Baked Salmon	1 salmon fillet	Lemon slices, dill, side of steamed broccoli
Grilled Chicken	1 grilled chicken breast	Quinoa, roasted vegetables, a squeeze of lime
Stir-Fry	Mixed Vegetables	Tofu or lean beef, soy sauce, brown rice
Veggie Pasta	Whole grain pasta	Marinara sauce, sautéed zucchini, bell peppers
Stuffed Peppers	Bell peppers	Ground turkey, black beans, corn, quinoa

Dessert Options

Option	Base	Toppings/Extras
Fruit Salad	Mixed fresh fruits	Mint leaves, a squeeze of lime
Dark Chocolate	1-2 squares dark chocolate	Mixed berries
Chia Pudding	1 cup chia pudding	Fresh mango slices, coconut flakes
Baked Apple	1 baked apple	Cinnamon, a dollop of Greek yogurt
Yogurt with Honey	1 cup non-fat Greek yogurt	Drizzle of honey, sliced almonds

Beverage Options

Option	Base	Toppings/Extras
Green Tea	1 cup green tea	Lemon wedge, mint leaves
Infused Water	Water	Cucumber slices, fresh mint, lemon slices
Smoothie	1 cup almond milk	Spinach, banana, blueberries, flax seeds
Herbal Tea	1 cup herbal tea	Honey, lemon slice
Sparkling Water	Sparkling water	Splash of cranberry juice, lime wedge

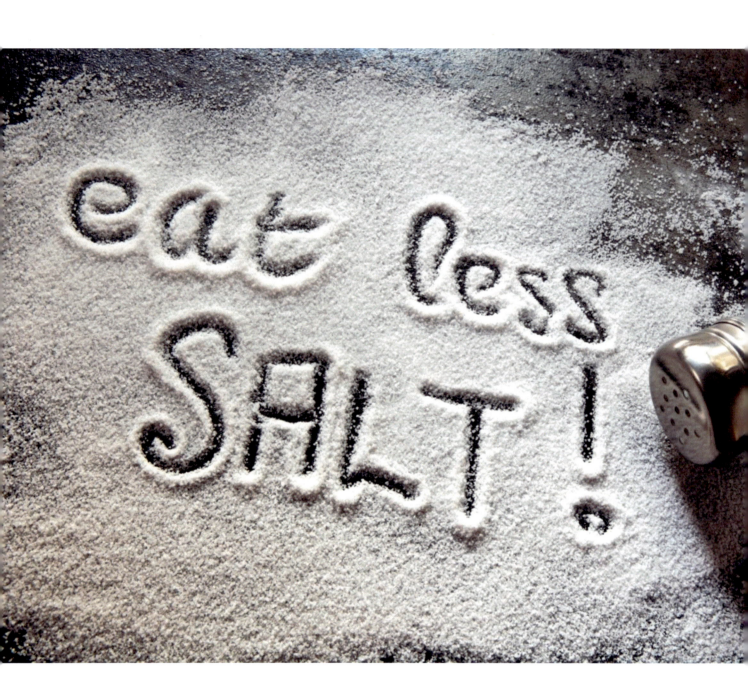

11.1.TECHNIQUES TO REDUCE FAT AND SODIUM

Reducing fat and sodium in your diet can be very important in improving your cardiovascular health and preventing chronic diseases. Demonstrating these components' powerful impact on health parameters has called nutritionists and other health professionals to design and refine techniques to restrict their use. So, what are the best techniques to reduce fat and sodium in our food?

Understanding Nutrition Labels:

Nutrition labeling on any package can be very useful in making an educated decision about food selection. The nutrition label gives details of the fat, sodium, and sugar content in the food item, helping one compare products and pick the healthier choice. Note also that serving size and the number of serving sizes per container should be checked to determine exactly how many nutrients may be consumed since the "total" values only estimate the given nutrient. Thus, one should compare the numbers for fat, sodium, and sugar across different products to pick a healthier choice that supports heart-healthy goals. For example, you can find a product sold with its saturated fat levels lowered, or you may purchase the low sodium variety of a particular food product. Second, nutrition labels may aid you in monitoring your total calorie intake, which is significant in connection with your ability to control your weight and reduce your chance of heart-related issues linked to being overweight.

Choosing Lean Proteins:

Incorporating lean proteins into your Heart healthy diet is a crucial step in the direction of retaining a healthy heart. These protein resources are not only low in saturated fat but also provide vital vitamins that support usual cardiovascular health. When it comes to lean meats, chicken and turkey are exceptional selections as they may be obviously low in saturated fats and excessive in protein. Additionally, fish, specifically fatty fish like salmon and mackerel, provide a completely unique source of lean protein and coronary heart-healthy omega-3 fatty acids.

Numerous research studies have highlighted the benefits of omega-3 fatty acids in decreasing the threat of heart disorders. These types of fat have been proven to lower triglyceride degrees, lessen irritation, and prevent blood clots, all of which contribute to a healthier cardiovascular system. Regularly incorporating lean proteins like those into your meals ensures you get the essential vitamins while heading off the dangers of high saturated fat intake.

Increasing Fruits and Vegetables:

Fruits and greens are the cornerstones of a healthy heart diet program. These nutrient-dense ingredients are full of dietary fiber, nutrients, and minerals that can help assist cardiovascular fitness. The fiber observed in results and veggies facilitates the adjustment of cholesterol levels and healthy digestion. At the same time, nutrients and minerals play essential roles in numerous physical features and in maintaining a healthy heart. One of the most crucial benefits of increasing your fruit and vegetable consumption is their low-calorie and genuinely healthy fat nature. By incorporating a broad type of colorful fruits and vegetables into your food, you will nourish your body with vital vitamins and prevent heart diseases. Furthermore, colorful fruits and vegetables are characterized by being high in phytochemical proprieties. These plant compounds, which include flavonoids and carotenoids, have been shown to possess mighty antioxidant and anti-inflammatory characteristics that may help protect the heart and blood vessels from oxidative strain and irritation-associated harm.

Limit Foods High in Fat:

Not all fats are harmful, but high-fat foods, particularly those with saturated fat, must be limited. These include red meat, cheese, and baked foods, which cause heart diseases due to high cholesterol levels. Saturated fats also increase the levels of low-density lipoprotein, the "bad" cholesterol, in the body. This may result in the narrowing of arteries, which will eventually restrict blood flow and cause an increased number of heart attacks and strokes. One can reduce consumption of saturated fats by not eating high-fat foods and, alternatively, consuming low-fat foods such as plant meals or lean meat cuts. Such a move in diet will decrease the number of LDL cholesterols and eventually lead to an effective cardiovascular system.

Limit High-Sodium Foods:

Too much sodium is one of the leading causes of hypertension, which is among the significant factors that lead to heart disease. Most processed foods, such as sandwiches, pizza, soups, and snacks, are high in salt. It is incredibly vital to be aware of your sodium intake. High blood pressure strains the heart and blood vessels, raising the risk of heart attacks, strokes, and other cardiovascular complications. You can consume much less sodium, which may help lower blood pressure, by eating less high-sodium foods and choosing fresh or home-cooked options with lots of herbs and spices for flavor. And remember, the saltshaker isn't the only place sodium lurks; much hides in processed and packaged food items. Reading nutrition labels and being mindful of sodium content is a crucial step that will help you make informed decisions and feel confident in your food choices for the good of your heart.

Different ways of preparing the food:

Different ways of preparing food could mean a world of difference regarding nutritional value and whether it can be included in a heart-healthy diet. Use healthier methods and techniques in cooking, which in turn will cut down unhealthy fats and sodium but maintain natural flavors and nutrients of ingredients. Simple but effective is to trim visible fat from meats before cooking. If needed, these simple steps would easily cut your intake of saturated fat – which means less cholesterol and a healthier cardiovascular system. As an alternative to deep-frying or pan-frying, cooking your food by baking, grilling, or steaming doesn't add many extra calories or unhealthy fats to your food. Such preparation methods help you maintain the natural flavor of food without adding more fats or oils. Besides, one can always have fun with herbs, spices, and flavoring ingredients to add more dimension and excitement without using too much salt or unhealthy seasonings.

Wash Out Canned Foods:

Canned foods are cheap and convenient, but many contain added sodium for preservation. Rinsing canned beans and vegetables under running water can wash away as much as 40% of the sodium content, a minor procedure that could make them a healthier option for your meals. High sodium intake is associated with high blood pressure, an increased workload on the heart, and an associated raised risk of cardiovascular diseases. By rinsing canned foods before use, you'll significantly lower your sodium intake while still enjoying the convenience and economy of such products. It would be best to consider other nutritional values in the canned foods you go for. Select canned vegetables without added sauces or seasonings and canned beans or legumes that are low in sodium or labeled "no salt added."

Make partial switches:

If you are accustomed to consuming large amounts of regular, higher-sodium versions of food, gradual substitutions for the lower-sodium version will be beneficial. One great idea is mixing foods of the same food item but of a regular and lower-sodium version. It gives your taste buds time to adjust because they can be introduced slowly to the new changes. For example, you may want to try mixing half of a regular can with half of a low-sodium version if you often use a regular canned soup. As your taste buds adapt, you can gradually increase the lower-sodium product amount until you no longer feel the need for the other product. This may also be true for bread, sauces, and condiments. Reduce progressively your sodium; you're less likely to miss it and more likely to stick with a heart-healthy diet.

Note:

Just remember, everyone is unique, and their tastes and diet needs vary, so please consult with your healthcare professional or a registered dietitian when developing a personal plan that will meet your exact requirements and goals for heart health.

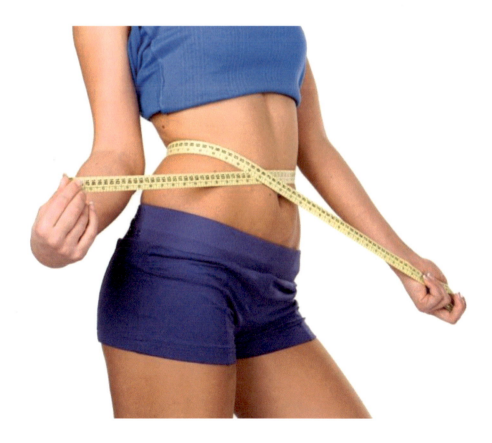

11.2. USING HERBS AND SPICES TO ENHANCE FLAVOR

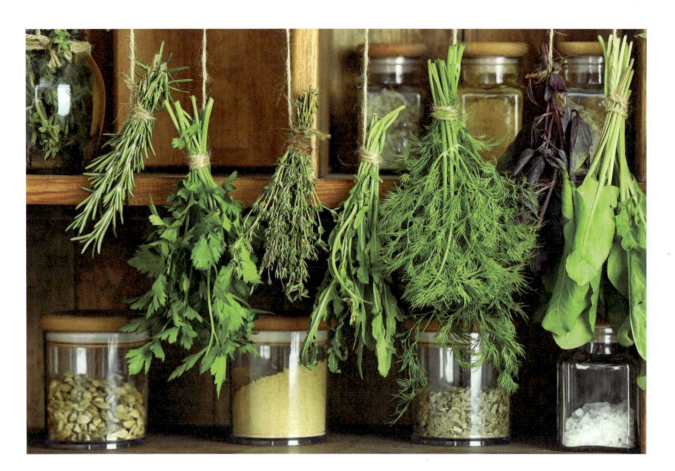

"**H**erbs and spices are the friends of physicians and precious jewels for the choice of life, sparkling like the radiant blossoms of spring." —Pliny the Elder, AD 23–79, a Roman naturalist and philosopher. The above quote says it all: how herbs and spices season our food best and cater to healthier eating. Pliny the Elder counted these natural ingredients as very good for cooking and a healthy life. And this is where herbs and spices come in like magic. They are the perfect way to bump up the taste in your heart-healthy diet without all the extra salt, sugar, or unhealthy fats. Using a variety of herbs and spices in your cooking will bring out your taste and, at the same time, help you benefit from their wide-ranging health advantages. These natural flavor enhancers can add to the general sensory experience of eating, making it satisfying and pleasurable.

Experiment with fresh herbs—basil, cilantro, parsley, rosemary, thyme, and mint: Fresh herbs add a burst of freshness to everything they come into contact with. Their vibrant flavors are ideal for uplifting salads, soups, and pasta. Fresh herbs are not only for the pleasure of the palette; they are loaded with antioxidants and vitamins that aid digestion and are sources of anti-inflammatory support.

Besides, dried herbs and spices are pantry staples and magic ingredients that add concentrated flavor to any dish. They are wonderfully versatile and can be put in a dish at any cooking stage. Cumin adds earthiness to a stew; paprika lends a sweet piquancy to meats, and turmeric has a warm bitterness. Cinnamon adds sweetness to desserts, garlic powder boosts savoriness, and onion powder augments its flavor with a subtle sharpness. Anything will be livened up with adding chili powder to add spice. Moreover, mixing different herbs and spices enables one to have made-to-order herb and spice mixtures that suit one's taste. An Italian blend might contain oregano, basil, rosemary, and garlic powder, for instance, and it's perfect for a pasta sauce or the topping for a pizza. A Moroccan blend might contain cumin, coriander, cinnamon, and ginger and be ideal for adding to a tagine or couscous.

We can also add herbs and spices as a rub or marinade. Indeed, protein and marinades are a great way to get flavor into your food. A little garlic, paprika, and black pepper rub can spice up grilled chicken. A lemon-herb marinade can give fish fillets a refreshing tang. And we don't forget to use aromatic vegetables like onions, garlic, ginger, and chili, which are the essential ingredients upon which layers of flavor are built in cooking. By sautéing these aromatics at the beginning of a recipe, their essential oils are set free to create a base that enhances the dish's overall flavor.

We can incorporate herbs and spices into sauces and dressings. For instance, herbs and spices in a sauce or dressing can add flavor. You can also make your pesto with basil, pine nuts, or garlic. Use it as a versatile sauce for pasta or sandwiches—herbed vinaigrette with Dijon mustard for salads or as a marinade. Roasting vegetables caramelizes their natural sugars and intensifies their flavors. Toss them with olive oil, herbs, and spices before roasting for additional flavor depth. We can flavor Grains and Legumes. Grains such as quinoa, rice, barley, and legumes such as lentils and beans are healthy-based foods that enhance flavor by adding herbs and spices. They take on flavors well and can be transformed from bland to grand with the proper seasoning. They are readily prepared yet offer great complex flavors for any dish. Drizzle a little on top of a caprese salad with basil-infused olive oil, use rosemary-infused vinegar in a marinade, and add subtle but distinct notes to your cooking. In short, better heart health is another advantage of embracing the natural flavors of herbs and spices in your cooking routine.

11.3. COOKING METHODS THAT PRESERVE NUTRIENTS

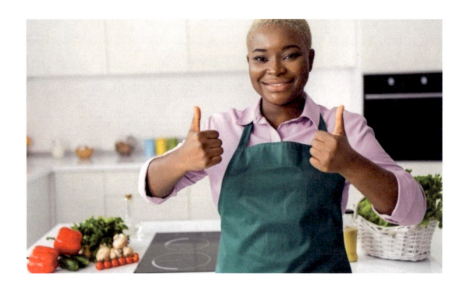

The nutrient value of foods can be retained through proper cooking methods that do not destroy food. Different cooking methods affect food nutrients differently. So, let's see in more detail each process and how it helps in nutrient preservation:

Steaming: It ranks among the top techniques for nutrient preservation. This method involves cooking food over fast-flowing boiling water in a covered pot or steamer. Since the food does not come into direct contact with water, which would result in a loss of nutrients, the gentle cooking effect of steam is employed. Vegetables, fish, and meats can be effectively cooked using this method. The relatively short cooking process helps preserve some essential water-soluble vitamins, such as C and B, crucial to overall health.

Microwaving: This is a cooking method where food is cooked evenly and fast due to electromagnetic waves. It uses a small quantity of water in the cooking process, therefore leaching fewer nutrients compared to methods where foods are cooked in a large volume of water. Rapid cooking helps to preserve heat-sensitive nutrients, like vitamin C and some antioxidants, which are degraded by long periods of exposure to heat.

Sous Vide: The gentle process of sous vide involves vacuum-sealing food and cooking it underwater at exactly low temperatures for an extended period. The sous vide technique is more appropriate for recovering sensitive nutrients from heat and oxidants. Ideal for meats and fish, sous vide retains moisture and flavor, holds vitamins, and makes this the way chefs would prefer to keep food of high quality.

Stir-frying: It is the quick cooking of food in a small amount of oil over moderately high heat, which lowers nutrient loss, especially for those sensitive to heat, like vitamin C and B vitamins. Vegetables cooked by this method are bright in color and crisp in texture; less nutrient loss is evident here compared to other cooking processes.

Grilling/Broiling: This fast method of cooking food at high temperatures retains most of the nutrients. However, drippings from meat can lead to some nutrient loss, and charred parts may contain potentially harmful compounds. Meats can be marinated pre-cooking to counteract this process and should be turned frequently while cooking.

Baking/Roasting: By cooking food in an oven at moderate or high heat levels, baking and roasting help develop flavors without the need for abundant water. There is little loss of nutrients with this process, but, once again, it is better than boiling as less water is used. One needs to employ minimal cooking oils and wrap the food in foil or lids to retain the nutrients.

Blanching: This method involves quickly plunging the food into boiling water and then immersing it in ice-cold water to stop cooking. This method is primarily used for vegetables and is very efficient in retaining their color, structure, and nutrients. Compared to boiling, where nutrients leach into the water, blanching reduces this; hence, it is an exemplary method of maintaining nutrients.

Pressure Cooking: This method cooks food quickly through steam and high pressure, reducing cooking time and food exposure to oxygen and water. It is, therefore, perfect for beans, grains, and tougher meat because it retains more vitamins and minerals than boiling or simmering over a longer period.

Slow cooking: Slow cooking involves cooking with low heat over a long period; it is, therefore, well known for preserving flavors and textures. While it may cause some nutrient loss due to extended cooking times, more significant vegetable cuts and adding delicate ingredients towards the end can help minimize this effect.

Raw or Minimal Cooking: Eating raw or minimally cooked foods is ideal for preserving nutrients because they are not exposed to heat. However, not all foods are suitable to eat raw due to safety concerns or palatability. For ingredients inappropriate for raw consumption, cooking is the least possible way to preserve the most nutrients in the food.

Note:
In short, the cooking technique determines the nutrient content of the food. Cooking methods such as steaming, microwaving, sous vide, and stir-frying are more nutrient-rich than boiling or frying. By fusing different techniques, cooking timings, and heating temperatures, one can get the most out of the nutrients in the foods one eats for excellent health and well-being.

11.4. LONG-TERM DIETARY ADJUSTMENTS

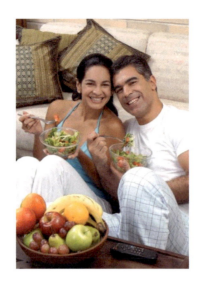

Adopting a heart-healthy dietary pattern requires diligence and patience, but the payoffs are boundless. Within this core structure of long-term dietary adjustments, building a deep understanding of the complicated interrelations between the food we eat and our cardiovascular system's health stands out. After all, a heart-healthy diet is not just a change in what we eat but a deeper appreciation of nutrition's role in our overall health and vitality. This journey begins with the great exploration of nutrient-rich foods, more so those rich in potassium, which plays a significant role in controlling blood pressure. It counterbalances the effect of sodium and removes tension from the walls of blood vessels—pivotal in the way it helps maintain healthy blood pressure. Among the foods that contain the most potassium are leafy greens such as spinach and kale, beans and lentils, and many brightly colored fruits and vegetables, such as bananas, oranges, and sweet potatoes. These potassium-rich foods contain other essential nutrients, including fiber, vitamins, and antioxidants. All these components are necessary for the health of the cardiovascular system in general, reduction of inflammation, and protection from oxidative stress, which is constant and involves many challenges that put the human body to the test.

As we dive deeper into these transforming dietary changes, we find the deep affinity between dishes and their aromas and flavors. A hint of chili peppers warms the body, improves blood circulation, and boosts metabolism, whereas cumin and coriander have earthy undertones that favor digestion and are anti-inflammatory. Adding fresh herbs, such as cilantro and mint, will enhance aroma and make the dishes more revitalizing and refreshing. It is a beautiful culinary symphony that can awaken the senses, developing a deep appreciation for the beauty and diversity of our world's culinary tapestry. It certainly isn't just about the pleasures of taste; it's a sacred ritual that binds the physical and spiritual body and soul. Every bite, every flavor enjoyed in turn, is a balance between our very selves and this rich bounty that is the earth's. Each time we experience the taste, it acts as a reminder of the thousands of careful relationships through which we are tethered to the natural world and the flow of life that, always without failure, has had the capability of sustaining our presence. Eating becomes the act of mindfulness and gratitude towards the labor of the hands that grow, harvest, and prepare our food. Every forkful of roasted sweet potatoes—warmed with cumin and flavored with cilantro's earthy essence. This confluence of heat, aroma, and taste gives us if only for a few moments, a glimpse into the very heart of existence. This commitment to a healthier lifestyle and long-term dietary adjustments is a celebration of life that can strengthen our heart health. Here are a few critical adjustments for long-term nutritional modifications that can support a heart-healthy lifestyle:

Gradual and Sustainable Changes: Rather than trying abrupt dietary changes, it's regularly more effective to introduce slow modifications that may be difficult to integrate into your everyday day. Small, incremental steps are more likely to emerge as routine.

Portion Control and Mindful Eating: Besides healthy low-sodium meals, portion sizes are essential in preserving a balanced and heart-healthy diet. Practicing conscious eating, which includes paying attention to hunger and satiety cues, will let you expand a more healthy courting with meals and save you from overeating.

Meal Planning and Preparation: Dedicating time to planning and preparing nutrient-rich food could make it simpler to stick to a healthy heart weight loss plan. Meal prepping, batch cooking, and having healthy snacks can indeed help lessen the temptation to rely on unhealthy foods.

Involving Family and Friends: Making nutritional modifications as a family or regarding pals on your journey can provide treasured help and duty. Sharing heart-healthy recipes, cooking together, and inspiring each other could make the transition smoother and extra fun.

Dealing with Setbacks: It's essential to comprehend that setbacks that we can face are ordinary occurrences in any nutritional adventure. Instead of becoming discouraged, approach those situations with self-compassion and consider their possibilities to examine and refocus on your long-term goals.

Note:

Remember, a heart-healthy diet isn't always just a short-term period of restoration; it is a lifelong commitment to nourishing your body and lowering the threat of cardiovascular disease. It is only through making gradual, sustainable adjustments and seeking help while wishing that you can set up healthy adjustments that can improve your life.

CONCLUSION

As we end our journey through "Your Heart Healthy Cookbook for Beginners," it is clear that achieving and maintaining heart health is a lifestyle, not just a diet plan. This book has given you a play-by-play guide to living a heart-healthy life, with many delicious and nutritious recipes, tips, accurate and insightful facts about how to maintain a healthy heart, and facts that are practical and at hand. We have gone through the basics of a heart-healthy diet: understanding which nutrients your body cannot do without and coming up with easy ways of making healthy ingredient substitutions. We have successfully run away from that sticky issue of reading food labels, picking out the best ingredients to include in our meals while steering away from the ones that would be harmful to your heart.

The abundance of recipes in this book and their versatility ensures maintaining your food balanced and healthy; from invigorating starters and hearty breakfasts to delicious nibbles, interesting shakes, and sweet desserts, you have loads of great ideas to keep your diet diverse and engaging. This book has also included dishes satisfying different tastes and dietary needs: Whether it's a need for fish or omega-3-laden dishes, poultry recipes, vegetarian delights, or fresh vegetable side dishes, we have it all. In addition to the recipes, this book has armed you with expert tips for lifelong health. We've pooled the best nutritionist knowledge to help keep you motivated and make those essential adjustments to your diet while still enjoying flavor.

The 30-day meal plans and weekly shopping lists included in this book are a practical tool to get you started on the way back to health and help keep you on track. Finally, this book has also armed you with advanced cooking techniques that bring your culinary abilities to the next level: preparing foods in healthy and delicious ways. Fat and sodium reduction, advanced herb and spice usage, and retaining food nutrients by proper cooking methods—are all essential parts of a culinary toolkit.

Your heart is a lifelong journey. Waking up every day and including the information and recipes from this book in your daily routine is a significant investment in your health. Stick with it, get experimental in the kitchen, but most importantly, enjoy nurturing your heart with each meal you make.

This book will guide you to a future filled with great food, brilliant health, and endless possibilities. Choosing this road will lead you to a life of wellness and joy, so seize it.

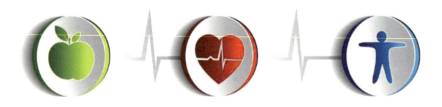

Made in the USA
Columbia, SC
17 April 2025

8ed4c892-3262-4ed5-9363-f1c38592015cR01